ANTI-INFLAMMATORY DIET FOR BEGINNERS

100 MOUTHWATERING RECIPES TO FIGHT INFLAMMATION, BOOST THE IMMUNE SYSTEM AND YOUR WEIGHT LOSS

ANTI-INFLAMMATORY DIET FOR BEGINNERS

© Copyright 2021 - All rights reserved.

The content contained within this book may not be reproduced, duplicated or transmitted without direct written permission from the author or the publisher. Under no circumstances will any blame or legal responsibility be held against the publisher, or author, for any damages, reparation, or monetary loss due to the information contained within this book. Either directly or indirectly.

Legal Notice:

This book is copyright protected. This book is only for personal use. You cannot amend, distribute, sell, use, quote or paraphrase any part, or the content within this book, without the consent of the author or publisher.

Disclaimer Notice:

Please note the information contained within this document is for educational and entertainment purposes only. All effort has been executed to present accurate, up to date, and reliable, complete information. No warranties of any kind are declared or implied. Readers acknowledge that the author is not engaging in the rendering of legal, financial, medical or professional advice. The content within this book has been derived from various sources. Please consult a licensed professional before attempting any techniques outlined in this book.

By reading this document, the reader agrees that under no circumstances is the author responsible for any losses, direct or indirect, which are incurred as a result of the use of information contained within this document, including, but not limited to, errors, omissions, or inaccuracies.

Table of Contents

INTRODUCTION 8
    Symptoms of Inflammation 9
    Foods to Eat 10
    Foods to Avoid 11

CHAPTER 1: BREAKFAST 12
1. Leek & Spinach Frittata 13
2. Cherry Chia Oats 14
3. Oven-Poached Eggs 15
4. Cranberry and Raisins Granola 16
5. Spicy Marble Eggs 17
6. Gingerbread Oatmeal Breakfast 18
7. Apple, Ginger, and Rhubarb Muffins 19
8. Anti-Inflammatory Breakfast Frittata 20
9. Breakfast Sausage and Mushroom Casserole 21
10. Cheesy Flax and Hemp Seeds Muffins 22
11. Fantastic Spaghetti Squash with Cheese and Basil Pesto 23
12. Flaxseed Porridge with Cinnamon 24
13. Breakfast Pitas 25
14. Shirataki Pasta with Avocado and Cream 26
15. Cinnamon Pancakes with Coconut 27
16. Yummy Steak Muffins 28
17. Nutty Oats Pudding 29
18. Banana Pancakes 30
19. Baked French Toast Casserole 31
20. Whole Grain Blueberry Scones 32

CHAPTER 2: SNACKS, SIDES, AND APPETIZERS 34
1. Creamy Polenta 35
2. Mushroom Millet 36
3. Roasted Curried Cauliflower 37
4. Caramelized Pears and Onions 38
5. Spicy Roasted Brussels Sprouts 39
6. Apple Sauce Treat 40
7. Brownies Avocado 41
8. Brussels Sprout Chips 42
9. Cauliflower Snacks 43
10. Ginger Flour Banana Ginger Bars 44

11.	Tangy Turmeric Flavored Florets	45
12.	Cool Garbanzo and Spinach Beans	46
13.	Onion and Orange Healthy Salad	47
14.	Oven Crisp Sweet Potato	48
15.	Olive and Tomato Balls	49
16.	Stir-Fried Almond and Spinach	50
17.	Cilantro and Avocado Platter	51
18.	Spicy Barley	52
19.	Tender Farro	53
20.	Wheatberry Salad	54

CHAPTER 3: LUNCH 56

1.	Pan-Seared Scallops with Lemon-Ginger Vinaigrette	57
2.	Manhattan-Style Salmon Chowder	58
3.	Sesame-Tuna Skewers	59
4.	Trout with Chard	60
5.	Seafood Noodles	61
6.	Spicy Pulled Chicken Wraps	62
7.	Apricot Chicken Wings	63
8.	Champion Chicken Pockets	64
9.	Chicken-Bell Pepper Sauté	65
10.	Curried Beef Meatballs	66
11.	Beef Meatballs in Tomato Gravy	67
12.	Pork with Lemongrass	68
13.	Pork with Olives	69
14.	Avocado-Orange Grilled Chicken	70
15.	Honey Chicken Tagine	71
16.	Potato Dumpling with Shrimp	72
17.	Shrimp Rissoles	73
18.	Sole with Vegetables	74
19.	Roasted Salmon and Asparagus	75
20.	Citrus Salmon on a Bed of Greens	76
21.	Orange and Maple-Glazed Salmon	77

CHAPTER 4: DINNER 78

1.	Lemony Mussels	79
2.	Hot Tuna Steak	80
3.	Marinated Fish Steaks	81
4.	Baked Tomato Hake	82
5.	Healthy Fish Nacho Bowl	83
6.	Buffalo Chicken Lettuce Wraps	84

7.	Cilantro-Lime Chicken Drumsticks	85
8.	Coconut-Curry-Cashew Chicken	86
9.	Turkey & Sweet Potato Chili	87
10.	Moroccan Turkey Tagine	88
11.	Parsley Pork and Artichokes	89
12.	Pork with Mushrooms and Cucumbers	90
13.	Oregano Pork	91
14.	Creamy Pork and Tomatoes	92
15.	Pork with Balsamic Onion Sauce	93
16.	Ground Pork Pan	94
17.	Fish & Chickpea Stew	95
18.	Duck Legs and Wine Sauce	96
19.	Chicken Piccata	97
20.	Honey-Mustard Lemon Marinated Chicken	98
21.	Easy Crunchy Fish Tray Bake	99
22.	Ginger & Chili Sea Bass Fillets	100
23.	Cheesy Tuna Pasta	101
24.	Salmon and Roasted Peppers	102

CHAPTER 5: DESSERTS 104

1.	Chocolate Chip Quinoa Granola Bars	104
2.	Sherbet Pineapple	105
3.	Easy Peach Cobbler	106
4.	Thar She Salts Peanut Butter Cookies	107
5.	Fruit Cobbler	108
6.	Watermelon and Avocado Cream	109
7.	Coconut and Chocolate Cream	110
8.	Chocolate Bananas	111
9.	Watermelon Sorbet	112
10.	Almond Butter Balls Vegan	113
11.	Coffee Cream	114
12.	Almond Cookies	115
13.	Chocolate Mousse	116
14.	Strawberry Granita	117
15.	Apple Fritters	118

CONCLUSION 120

Introduction

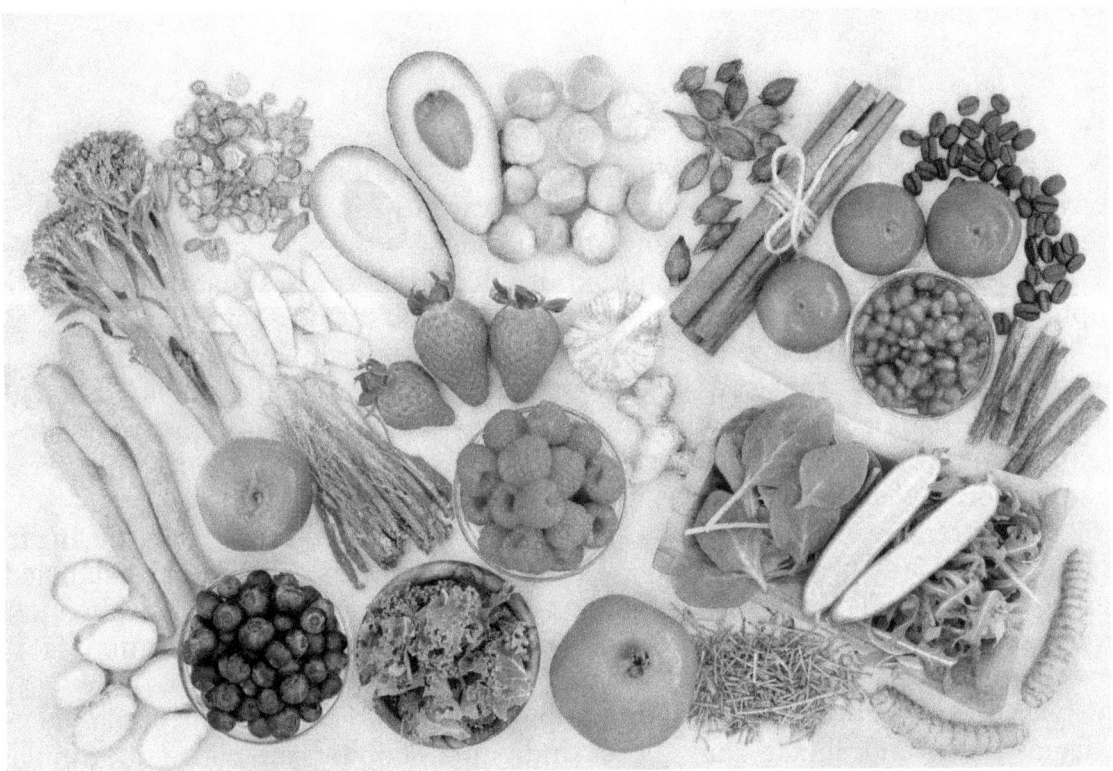

The anti-inflammatory diet is not just for weight loss, although you may lose weight while on this diet. It is not a limited, three-week trek to push current inflammation from the body. It is not a false, quick leap to health. It provides a specific, new approach to your life: a way of life complete with all the nutrients and minerals, calories, and proteins that one needs to live well and happily. The anti-inflammatory diet components will help boost your overall health by providing the necessary nutrients and inflammation-fighting compounds to allow your body to heal itself and maintain proper balance. You will begin to notice changes in how you look and feel. You will have a sense of renewed energy. Your skin will take on an unmistakable healthy glow. Your body will be working correctly, producing new healthy cells, and calming the chaos of inflammation within your system. To follow the anti-inflammatory diet and reap the health benefits, you must understand yourself.

Symptoms of Inflammation

The main signs of inflammation include; heat, redness, pain, swelling, and muscle-function loss. These symptoms depend on the inflamed body part and its cause. Some of the widespread signs of chronic inflammation are:
- Frequent infections.
- Weight gain.
- Body pain.
- Insomnia.
- Fatigue.
- Mood disorders like anxiety and depression.
- Gastrointestinal problems like diarrhea, constipation, and acid reflux disease.

The typical symptoms of inflammation rely on various inflammatory effect problems. When the body's defense mechanism, which influences the skin, causes rashes. When you are dealing with arthritis rheumatoid, it affects the joints. Most of the signs and symptoms experienced are fatigue, tingling, joint pains, stiffness, and swelling.

Similarly, when experiencing inflammatory bowel, it typically influences the digestive system. Its usual signs consist of bleeding ulcers, anemia, weight loss, bloating, pains, diarrhea, and stomach pains. With multiple sclerosis, the condition occurs on the myelin sheath, which covers the nerve cells. Its signs consist of problems when passing out stool, double vision, blurred eyesight, fatigue, and cognitive issues.

If you encounter any of the symptoms and health problems, you could be suffering from inflammation. Many people link it to joint pains like arthritis, which can be signaled by swelling and aches. The problem is related to health problems, not just swollen joints. Nevertheless, all soreness is not bad. For instance, acute inflammation is vital throughout recovery from a twisted and puffy ankle.

It is easy to detect Chronic inflammation signs and causes. Insomnia, genetic predisposition, food intake, and other individual habits can cause it. Similarly, inflammation resulting from allergic may also develop in your gut.

Below are some of the possibilities that you may be having:
- If you always feel tired to the extent of not having enough sleep, not getting enough nap, or sleeping excessively.
- Do you experience time-to-time aches and pains? It may also signify that you have arthritis.
- Are you experiencing any pain in the gut or stomachache? The pain may create inflammation. Gut inflammation may also cause cramping, bloating, and loose stools.
- A swollen lymph node is another sign of inflammation. These nodes lie in the neck, armpits, and groin, which swell if there is a problem in your system. When you have a sore throat, your neck nodes lump because the body's defense system has sensed the condition. These lymph nodes react since the body is fighting the infection. The nodes reshape as you heal.

- Is your nose stuffed up? If indeed, maybe it is a symptom of irritating nasal tooth cavities.
- Sometimes, your epidermis may protrude because of internal inflammation.

Foods to Eat

If you already eat an appropriate healthy diet, you will have no trouble incorporating these foods into your meals. You may already be enjoying them and need a few tweaks to increase their presence in your meal planning. Some of the right foods that prevent and reduce chronic inflammation are as follows:

Omega-3 Fatty Acids

Omega-3 fatty acids are found in fish and fish oil. They calm the white blood cells and help them realize there is no danger to return to dormancy. Wild salmon and other fish are good sources; it is recommended to eat them three times a week. Other foods rich in Omega-3s are flax meal and dry beans such as navy beans, kidney beans, and soybeans. An Omega-3 supplement may be helpful if you are not able to ingest enough of these foods.

Fruits and Vegetables

Most fruits and vegetables are anti-inflammatory. They are naturally rich in antioxidants, carotenoids, lycopene, and magnesium. Dark green leafy vegetables and colorful fruits and berries do much to inhibit white blood cell activity.

Protective Oils and Fats

Yes, there are a few oils and fats that are good for chronic inflammation sufferers. They include coconut oil and extra virgin olive oil. Butter or cream is also acceptable to consume. Ghee, made from butter, is even better because it has the lactose and casein removed—the very ingredients cause so much trouble if you have lactose intolerance or wheat sensitivity.

Fiber

Fiber keeps waste moving through the body. Since the vast majority of our immune cells reside in the intestines, it is essential to keep your gut happy. If that doesn't provide enough fiber, feel free to take a fiber supplement.

Miscellaneous

Eat foods with spices and herbs instead of bad fats and unsafe oils. Spices like turmeric, cumin, cloves, ginger, and cinnamon can enhance white blood cells' calming. Herbs like fennel, rosemary, sage, and thyme also reduce inflammation while adding delicious new flavors to your food.

Fermented foods like sauerkraut, buttermilk, yogurt, and kimchi contain helpful bacteria that prevent inflammation.

Healthy snacks would include a limited amount of unsweetened, plain yogurt with fruit mixed in, celery, carrots, pistachios, almonds, walnuts, and other fruits and vegetables.

Foods to Avoid

While many foods should be included in your diet to aid in reducing chronic inflammation, there are also some foods that you must avoid to help keep the inflammation down.

Processed foods and sugars are two of the biggest culprits when it comes to inflammation in the western diet. Processed foods are highly refined, causing them to lose much of their natural fiber and nutrients. They are often high in omega-6, trans fats, and saturated fats, increasing inflammation.

Sugar is one of the worst offenders when it comes to increased inflammation. Not only does it hide in many foods, studies have found that it is also very addictive. Because of this, you should expect to go through a withdrawal phase when you remove it from your diet. It can often cause headaches, cravings, and sluggishness. Give yourself some time to allow your body to work through it. You don't have to remove natural sugars from your diet entirely, but you should work towards eating them a few times a week and at no more than one meal per day.

Most fried foods, especially deep-fried foods, should be avoided as well. Usually, they are cooked in processed oils or lard and are coated in a refined flour that promotes inflammation.

You will want to pay attention to foods known as nightshades. Nightshades can be anti-inflammatory, but some people are sensitive to them; if you find you seem to have more inflammation after consuming nightshade, you may want to begin to make substitutions in your recipes.

CHAPTER 1:

Breakfast

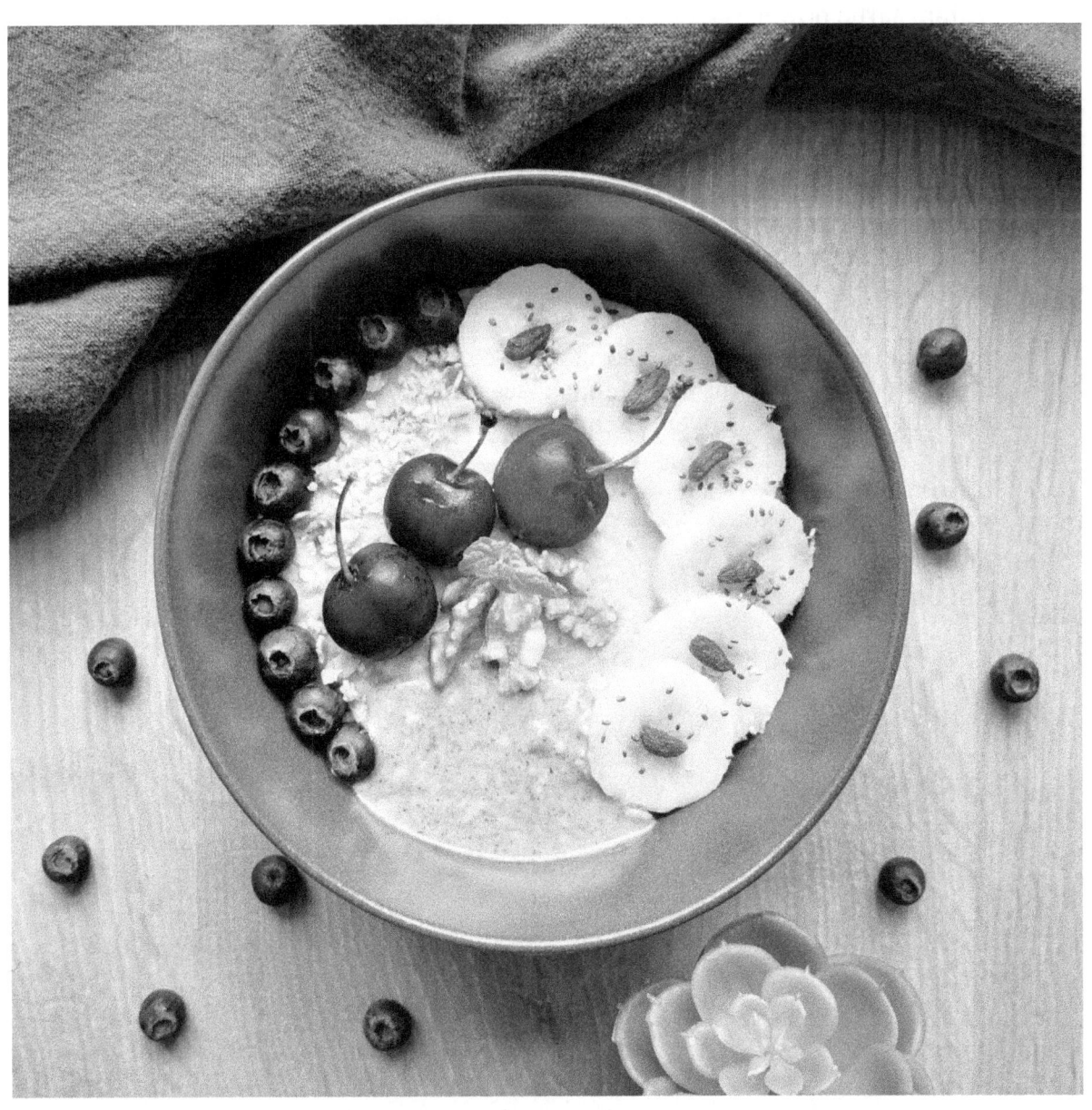

1. Leek & Spinach Frittata

Preparation Time: 10 minutes
Cooking Time: 15 minutes
Servings: 4
Ingredients:
- 2 leeks, chopped fine
- 2 tbsps. avocado oil
- 8 eggs
- ½ tsp. garlic powder
- ½ tsp. basil, dried
- 1 cup baby spinach, fresh & packed
- 1 cup cremini mushrooms, sliced
- Sea salt & black pepper to taste

Directions:
1. Set the oven to 400°F then get an oven-proof skillet. Place it over medium-high heat, sautéing your leeks in your avocado oil until soft. It should take roughly five minutes.
2. Get out a bowl, and whisk the eggs with your garlic, basil, and salt. Add them to the skillet with your leeks, cooking for five minutes. You'll need to stir frequently.
3. Stir in your mushrooms and spinach, seasoning with pepper.
4. Place the skillet in the oven, then bake for 10 minutes. Serve warm.

Nutrition:
- **Calories:** 276
- **Protein:** 19 g
- **Fat:** 17 g
- **Carbs:** 15 g

2. Cherry Chia Oats

Preparation Time: 10 minutes
Cooking Time: 20 minutes
Servings: 2
Ingredients:
- ¼ tsp. vanilla extract, pure
- 2 tbsps. almond butter
- 8 cherries, fresh, pitted, and halved
- 1 cup quick cook oats
- 2 tbsps. chia seeds
- ¼ cup whole milk yogurt, plain
- 1 ¼ cup almond milk

Directions:
1. Mix all the ingredients until they're combined well.
2. Seal in two jars and refrigerate for twenty-five minutes before serving.

Nutrition:
- **Calories:** 564
- **Protein:** 22 g
- **Fat:** 32 g
- **Carbs:** 27 g

3. Oven-Poached Eggs

Preparation Time: 2 minutes
Cooking Time: 11 minutes
Servings: 4
Ingredients:
- 6 eggs, at room temperature
- Water

Ice bath:
- 2 cups water, chilled
- 2 cups of ice cubes

Directions:
1. Set the oven to 350°F. Put 2 cups of water into a deep roasting tin, and place it into the lowest rack of the oven.
2. Place one egg into each cup of cupcake/muffin tins, along with one tbsp. water.
3. Carefully place muffin tins into the middle rack of the oven.
4. Bake eggs for 45 minutes.
5. Turn off the heat immediately. Take off the muffin tins from the oven and set them on a cake rack to cool before extracting eggs.
6. Pour ice bath ingredients into a large heat-resistant bowl.
7. Bring the eggs into an ice bath to stop the cooking process. After 10 minutes, drain the eggs well. Use as needed.

Nutrition:
- **Calories:** 357
- **Protein:** 17.14 g
- **Fat:** 24.36 g
- **Carbs:** 16.19 g

4. Cranberry and Raisins Granola

Preparation Time: 15 minutes
Cooking Time: 20 minutes
Servings: 4
Ingredients:
- 4 cups old-fashioned rolled oats
- 1/4 cup sesame seeds
- 1 cup dried cranberries
- 1 cup golden raisins
- 1/8 tsp. nutmeg
- 2 tbsps. olive oil
- 1/2 cup almonds, slivered
- 2 tbsps. warm water
- 1 tsp. vanilla extract
- 1 tsp. cinnamon
- 1/4 tsp. salt
- 6 tbsps. maple syrup
- 1/3 cup honey

Directions:
1. In a bowl, mix sesame seeds, nutmeg, almonds, oats, salt, and cinnamon.
2. In another bowl, mix oil, water, vanilla, honey, and syrup. Gradually pour the mixture into the oats mixture. Toss to combine. Spread the mixture into a greased jelly-roll pan. Bake in the oven at 300°F for at least 55 minutes. Stir and break the clumps every 10 minutes.
3. Once you get it from the oven, stir the cranberries and raisins. Allow cooling. This will last for a week when stored in an airtight container and up to a month when stored in the fridge.

Nutrition:
- **Calories:** 698
- **Protein:** 21.34 g
- **Fat:** 20.99 g
- **Carbs:** 148.59 g

5. Spicy Marble Eggs

Preparation Time: 15 minutes
Cooking Time: 2 hours
Servings: 12
Ingredients:
- 6 medium-boiled eggs, unpeeled, cooled

For the Marinade:
- 2 oolong black tea bags
- 3 tbsp. brown sugar
- 1 thumb-sized fresh ginger, unpeeled, crushed
- 3 dried star anise, whole
- 2 dried bay leaves
- 3 tbsp. light soy sauce
- 4 tbsp. dark soy sauce
- 4 cups water
- 1 dried cinnamon stick, whole
- 1 tsp. salt
- 1 tsp. dried Szechuan peppercorns

Directions:
1. Using the back of a metal spoon, crack eggshells in places to create a spider web effect. Do not peel. Set aside until needed.
2. Pour marinade into a large Dutch oven set over high heat. Put lid partially on. Bring water to a rolling boil, about 5 minutes. Turn off heat.
3. Secure lid. Steep ingredients for 10 minutes.
4. Using a slotted spoon, fish out and discard solids. Cool marinade completely to room proceeding.
5. Place eggs into an airtight non-reactive container just small enough to snugly fit all these in.
6. Pour in marinade. Eggs should be completely submerged in liquid. Discard leftover marinade, if any. Line container rim with generous layers of saran wrap. Secure container lid.
7. Chill eggs for 24 hours before using.
8. Extract eggs and drain each piece well before using, but keep the rest submerged in the marinade.

Nutrition:
- **Calories:** 75
- **Protein:** 4.05 g
- **Fat:** 4.36 g
- **Carbs:** 4.83 g

6. Gingerbread Oatmeal Breakfast

Preparation Time: 10 minutes
Cooking Time: 5 minutes
Servings: 4
Ingredients:
- 1 cup steel-cut oats
- 4 cups drinking water
- Organic Maple syrup, to taste
- 1 tsp ground cloves
- 1 ½ tbsp. ground cinnamon
- 1/8 tsp. nutmeg
- ¼ tsp. ground ginger
- ¼ tsp. ground coriander
- ¼ tsp. ground allspice
- ¼ tsp. ground cardamom
- Fresh mixed berries

Directions:
1. Cook the oats based on the package instructions. When it comes to a boil, reduce heat and simmer.
2. Stir in all the spices and continue cooking until cooked to desired doneness.
3. Serve in four serving bowls and drizzle with maple syrup and top with fresh berries.
4. Enjoy!

Nutrition:
- **Calories:** 87
- **Protein:** 5.82 g
- **Fat:** 3.26 g
- **Carbs:** 18.22 g

7. Apple, Ginger, and Rhubarb Muffins

Preparation Time: 15 minutes
Cooking Time: 25 minutes
Servings: 4
Ingredients:

- ½ cup finely ground almonds
- ¼ cup brown rice flour
- ½ cup buckwheat flour
- 1/8 cup unrefined raw sugar
- 2 tbsps. arrowroot flour
- 1 tbsp. linseed meal
- 2 tbsps. crystallized ginger, finely chopped
- ½ tsp. ground ginger
- ½ tsp. ground cinnamon
- 2 tsps. gluten-free baking powder
- A pinch of fine sea salt
- 1 small apple, peeled and finely diced
- 1 cup finely chopped rhubarb
- 1/3 cup almond/ rice milk
- 1 large egg
- ¼ cup extra virgin olive oil
- 1 tsp. pure vanilla extract

Directions:

1. Set your oven to 350°F, grease an eight-cup muffin tin, and line with paper cases.
2. Combine the almond four, linseed meal, ginger, and sugar in a mixing bowl. Sieve this mixture over the other flours, spices, and baking powder and use a whisk to combine well.
3. Stir in the apple and rhubarb in the flour mixture until evenly coated.
4. In a separate bowl, whisk the milk, vanilla, and egg, then pour it into the dry mixture. Stir until just combined—don't overwork the batter as this can yield very tough muffins.
5. Scoop the mixture into the arranged muffin tin and top with a few slices of rhubarb. Bake for at least 25 minutes, till they start turning golden or when an inserted toothpick emerges clean.
6. Take off from the oven and let sit for at least 5 minutes before transferring the muffins to a wire rack for further cooling.
7. Serve warm with a glass of squeezed juice.
8. Enjoy!

Nutrition:

- **Calories:** 325 **Protein:** 6.32 g **Fat:** 9.82 g **Carbs:** 55.71 g

8. Anti-Inflammatory Breakfast Frittata

Preparation Time: 10 minutes
Cooking Time: 40 minutes
Servings: 4
Ingredients:
- 4 large eggs
- 6 egg whites
- 450 g button mushrooms
- 450 g baby spinach
- 125 g firm tofu
- 1 onion, chopped
- 1 tbsp. minced garlic
- ½ tsp. ground turmeric
- ½ tsp. cracked black pepper
- ¼ cup water
- Kosher salt to taste

Directions:
1. Set your oven to 350°F.
2. Sauté the mushrooms in a little bit of extra virgin olive oil in a large non-stick oven-proof pan over medium heat. Add the onions once the mushrooms start turning golden and cook for 3 minutes until the onions become soft.
3. Stir in the garlic, then cook for at least 30 seconds until fragrant before adding the spinach. Pour in water, cover, and cook until the spinach becomes wilted for about 2 minutes.
4. Take off the lid and continue cooking up until the water evaporates. Now, combine the eggs, egg whites, tofu, pepper, turmeric, and salt in a bowl. When all the liquid has evaporated, pour in the egg mixture, let cook for about 2 minutes until the edges start setting, then transfer to the oven and bake for about 25 minutes or until cooked.
5. Take off from the oven then let sit for at least 5 minutes before cutting it into quarters and serving.
6. Enjoy!

Note: Baby spinach and mushrooms boost the nutrient profile of the eggs to provide you with amazing anti-inflammatory benefits.

Nutrition:
- **Calories:** 521
- **Protein:** 29.13 g
- **Fat:** 10.45 g
- **Carbs:** 94.94 g

9. Breakfast Sausage and Mushroom Casserole

Preparation Time: 20 minutes
Cooking Time: 45 minutes
Servings: 4
Ingredients:
- 450 g Italian sausage, cooked and crumbled
- 3/4 cup coconut milk
- 8 oz. white mushrooms, sliced
- 1 medium onion, finely diced
- 2 tbsps. organic ghee - 6 free-range eggs
- 600 g sweet potatoes - 1 red bell pepper, roasted
- 3/4 tsp. ground black pepper, divided
- 1 ½ tsp. sea salt, divided

Directions:
1. Peel and shred the sweet potatoes.
2. Take a bowl, fill it with ice-cold water, and soak the sweet potatoes in it. Set aside.
3. Peel the roasted bell pepper, remove its seeds and finely dice it.
4. Set the oven to 375°F.
5. Get a casserole baking dish and grease it with organic ghee.
6. Put a skillet over medium flame and cook the mushrooms in it. Cook until the mushrooms are crispy and brown.
7. Take the mushrooms out and mix them with the crumbled sausage.
8. Now sauté the onions in the same skillet. Cook up to the onions are soft and golden. This should take about 4–5 minutes.
9. Take the onions out and mix them in the sausage-mushroom mixture.
10. Add the diced bell pepper to the same mixture. Mix well and set aside for a while.
11. Now drain the soaked shredded potatoes, put them on a paper towel, and pat dry.
12. Bring the sweet potatoes to a bowl and add about a tsp. of salt and half a tsp. of ground black pepper to it. Mix well and set aside.
13. Now take a large bowl and crack the eggs in it. Break the eggs and then blend in the coconut milk. Stir in the remaining black pepper and salt.
14. Take the greased casserole dish and spread the seasoned sweet potatoes evenly in the base of the dish. Next, spread the sausage mixture evenly in the dish.
15. Finally, spread the egg mixture. Now cover the casserole dish using a piece of aluminum foil. Bake for 20–30 minutes. To check if the casserole is baked properly, insert a tester in the middle of the casserole, and it should come out clean.
16. Uncover the casserole dish and bake it again, uncovered for 5–10 minutes, until the casserole is a little golden on the top. Allow it to cool for 10 minutes. Enjoy!

Nutrition:
- **Calories:** 598 **Protein:** 28.65 g **Fat:** 36.75 g **Carbs:** 48.01 g

10. Cheesy Flax and Hemp Seeds Muffins

Preparation Time: 5 minutes
Cooking Time: 30 minutes
Servings: 2
Ingredients:
- 1/8 cup flaxseeds meal
- ¼ cup raw hemp seeds
- ¼ cup almond meal
- Salt, to taste
- ¼ tsp. baking powder
- 3 organic eggs, beaten
- 1/8 cup nutritional yeast flakes
- ¼ cup cottage cheese, low-fat
- ¼ cup grated parmesan cheese
- ¼ cup scallion, sliced thinly
- 1 tbsp. olive oil

Directions:
1. Switch on the oven, then set it 360°F and let it preheat.
2. Meanwhile, take two ramekins, grease them with oil, and set them aside until required.
3. Take a medium bowl, add flaxseeds, hemp seeds, and almond meal, and then stir in salt and baking powder until mixed.
4. Crack eggs in another bowl, add yeast, cottage cheese, and parmesan, stir well until combined, and then stir this mixture into the almond meal mixture until incorporated.
5. Fold in scallions, then distribute the mixture between prepared ramekins and bake for 30 minutes until muffins are firm and the top is nicely golden brown.
6. When done, take out the muffins from the ramekins and let them cool completely on a wire rack.
7. For meal prepping, wrap each muffin with a paper towel and refrigerate for up to thirty-four days.
8. When ready to eat, reheat muffins in the microwave until hot and then serve.

Nutrition:
- **Calories:** 179
- **Total Fat:** 10.9 g
- **Total Carbs:** 6.9 g
- **Protein:** 15.4 g
- **Sugar:** 2.3 g
- **Sodium:** 311 mg

11. Fantastic Spaghetti Squash with Cheese and Basil Pesto

Preparation Time: 10 minutes
Cooking Time: 35 minutes
Servings: 2

Ingredients:
- 1 cup cooked spaghetti squash, drained
- Salt, to taste
- Freshly cracked black pepper, to taste
- ½ tbsp. olive oil
- ¼ cup ricotta cheese, unsweetened
- 2 oz. fresh mozzarella cheese, cubed
- 1/8 cup basil pesto

Directions:
1. Switch on the oven, then set its temperature to 375°F and let it preheat.
2. Meanwhile, take a medium bowl, add spaghetti squash in it and then season with salt and black pepper.
3. Take a casserole dish, grease it with oil, add squash mixture in it, top it with ricotta cheese and mozzarella cheese and bake for 10 minutes until cooked.
4. When done, remove the casserole dish from the oven, drizzle pesto on top and serve immediately.

Nutrition:
- **Calories:** 169
- **Total Fat:** 11.3 g
- **Total Carbs:** 6.2 g
- **Protein:** 11.9 g
- **Sugar:** 0.1 g
- **Sodium:** 217 mg

12. Flaxseed Porridge with Cinnamon

Preparation Time: 10 minutes
Cooking Time: 5 minutes
Servings: 4
Ingredients:
- 1 tsp. cinnamon
- 1½ tsp. stevia
- 1 tbsp. unsalted butter
- 2 tbsp. flaxseed meal
- 2 tbsp. flaxseed oatmeal
- ½ cup shredded coconut
- 1 cup heavy cream
- 2 cups water

Directions:
1. Take a medium pot, place it over low heat, add all the ingredients in it, stir until mixed and bring the mixture to boil.
2. When the mixture has boiled, remove the pot from heat, stir it well and divide it evenly between four bowls.
3. Let porridge rest for 10 minutes until slightly thicken and then serve.

Nutrition:
- **Calories:** 171
- **Total Fat:** 16 g
- **Total Carbs:** 6 g
- **Protein:** 2 g

13. Breakfast Pitas

Preparation Time: 4 minutes
Cooking Time: 6 minutes
Servings: 4
Ingredients:
- 8 egg whites
- 2 cups bell peppers, chopped (any color)
- 1 tsp. garlic powder
- 1 tsp. onion powder
- 1 cup raw spinach (cook if you prefer)
- 2 tsps. extra virgin olive oil
- 4 whole-wheat pita pockets

Directions:
1. Put olive oil into a large sauté pan and place it over medium heat. When the oil is hot in glistening, toss in the bell pepper and sauté for about 3 minutes or until tender. Add in the spinach now (if you want it cooked) and sauté for about 1 to 3 minutes or just up to the sides starts to wilt.
2. Place the egg whites into a small bowl, whisk well. Add in spices; whisk well. Pour the egg mixture into the sauté pan and scramble everything together.
3. Remove from heat and stuff ½ to 1 cup mixture into a pita pocket and serve.

Nutrition:
- **Calories:** 153
- **Protein:** 12.4 g
- **Fat:** 3.41 g
- **Carbs:** 19.32 g

14. Shirataki Pasta with Avocado and Cream

Preparation Time: 10 minutes
Cooking Time: 6 minutes
Servings: 2

Ingredients:
- ½ packet shirataki noodles, cooked
- ½ avocado
- ½ tsp. cracked black pepper
- ½ tsp. salt
- ½ tsp. dried basil
- 1/8 cup heavy cream

Directions:
1. Place a medium pot half full with water over medium heat, bring it to boil, then add noodles and cook for 2 minutes.
2. Then drain the noodles and set them aside until required.
3. Place avocado in a bowl, mash it with a fork,
4. Mash avocado in a bowl, transfer it to a blender, add remaining ingredients, and pulse until smooth.
5. Take a frying pan, place it over medium heat and when hot, add noodles in it, pour in the avocado mixture, stir well and cook for 2 minutes until hot.
6. Serve straight away.

Nutrition:
- **Calories:** 131
- **Total Fat:** 12.6 g
- **Total Carbs:** 4.9 g
- **Protein:** 1.2 g
- **Sugar:** 0.3 g
- **Sodium:** 588 mg

15. Cinnamon Pancakes with Coconut

Preparation Time: 5 minutes
Cooking Time: 18 minutes
Servings: 2
Ingredients:
- 2 organic eggs
- 1 tbsp. almond flour
- 2 oz. cream cheese
- ¼ cup shredded coconut and more for garnishing
- ½ tbsp. erythritol
- 1/8 tsp. salt
- 1 tsp. cinnamon
- 4 tbsp. stevia
- ½ tbsp. olive oil

Directions:
1. Crack eggs in a bowl, beat until fluffy, and then beat in flour and cream cheese until smooth.
2. Add remaining ingredients and then stir until well combined.
3. Take a frying pan, place it over medium heat, grease it with oil, then pour in half of the batter and cook for 3 to 4 minutes per side until the pancake has cooked and nicely golden brown.
4. Transfer pancake to a plate and cook another pancake in the same manner by using the remaining batter.
5. Sprinkle coconut on top of cooked pancakes and serve.

Nutrition:
- **Calories:** 575
- **Total Fat:** 51 g
- **Total Carbs:** 3.5 g
- **Protein:** 19 g

16. Yummy Steak Muffins

Preparation Time: 10 minutes
Cooking Time: 20 minutes
Servings: 4
Ingredients:
- 1 cup red bell pepper, diced
- 2 Tbsps. water
- 8 oz. thin steak, cooked and finely chopped
- ¼ tsp. sea salt
- A dash of freshly ground black pepper
- 8 free-range eggs
- 1 cup finely diced onion

Directions:
1. Set the oven to 350°F
2. Take 8 muffin tins and line them with parchment paper liners.
3. Get a large bowl and crack all the eggs in it.
4. Beat well the eggs.
5. Blend in all the remaining ingredients.
6. Spoon the batter into the arranged muffin tins. Fill three-fourth of each tin.
7. Put the muffin tins in the preheated oven for about 20 minutes until the muffins are baked and set in the middle.
8. Enjoy!

Nutrition:
- **Calories:** 151
- **Protein:** 17.92 g
- **Fat:** 7.32 g
- **Carbs:** 3.75 g

17. Nutty Oats Pudding

Preparation Time: 10 minutes
Cooking Time: 3 minute
Servings: 3–5
Ingredients:
- ¼ cup rolled oats
- 1 tbsp. yogurt, fat-free
- 1 ½ tbsp. natural peanut butter
- ¼ cup dry milk
- 1 tsp. peanuts, finely chopped
- ½ cup water

Directions:
1. Using a microwaveable-safe bowl, put together peanut butter and dry milk. Whisk well. Add in water to achieve a smooth consistency. Add in oats.
2. Cover bowl with plastic wrap. Create a small hole for the steam to escape.
3. Place inside the microwave oven for 1 minute on high powder.
4. Continue heating, this time on medium power for 90 seconds. Let sit for 5 minutes.
5. To serve, spoon an equal amount of cereals in a bowl top with peanuts and yogurt.

Nutrition:
- **Calories:** 70
- **Protein:** 4.25 g
- **Fat:** 3.83 g
- **Carbs:** 6.78 g

18. Banana Pancakes

Preparation Time: 5 minutes
Cooking Time: 15 minutes
Servings: 2
Ingredients:
- 2 eggs
- 1 egg white
- 1 banana, ripe
- 1 cup rolled oats
- 2 tsps. ground cinnamon
- 1 tbsp. coconut oil, divided
- 1 tsp. vanilla extract, pure
- ½ tsp. sea salt

Directions:
1. Get out a food processor, grinding your oats until they make a coarse flour.
2. Add your cinnamon, egg whites, eggs, banana, vanilla, and salt. Blend until it forms a smooth batter and then heat a small skillet over medium heat. Heat half a tbsp. of coconut oil and then pour your batter in. Cook for two minutes per side and continue until all of your batter has been used.

Nutrition:
- **Calories:** 306
- **Protein:** 15 g
- **Fat:** 15 g
- **Carbs:** 17 g

19. Baked French Toast Casserole

Preparation Time: 20 minutes
Cooking Time: 45 minutes
Servings: 12
Ingredients:
- 1 lb. French bread
- 1 cup egg white liquid
- 6 eggs
- 1/3 cup maple syrup
- 1–1/2 cups rice milk
- ½ lb. raspberries
- ½ lb. blueberries
- 1 tsp. vanilla extract
- ¾ cup strawberries

Directions:
1. Slice the bread into small cubes. Keep them in a greased casserole dish.
2. Add all the berries. Only leave a few for the topping.
3. Whisk together the egg whites, eggs, rice milk, and vanilla extract in a bowl. Combine well.
4. Put the egg mixture on top of the bread. Press the bread down. All pieces should be soaked well.
5. Add berries on the top. Fill up the holes, if any.
6. Refrigerate covered for a couple of hours at least.
7. Take out the casserole half an hour before baking.
8. Set your oven to 350 degrees F.
9. Now, bake your casserole uncovered for 30 minutes.
10. Bake for another 15 minutes covered with a foil.
11. Let it rest for 15 minutes.
12. Serve it warm with maple syrup.

Nutrition:
- **Calories:** 200
- **Carbs:** 31 g
- **Cholesterol:** 93 mg
- **Total Fat:** 4 g
- **Protein:** 10 g
- **Fiber:** 2 g
- **Sodium:** 288 mg
- **Sugar:** 10 g

20. Whole Grain Blueberry Scones

Preparation Time: 10 minutes
Cooking Time: 25 minutes
Servings: 8
Ingredients:

- 2 cups whole-wheat flour
- ¼ cup maple syrup
- 6 tbsps. of olive oil
- 2-1/2 tsps. baking powder
- ½ tsp. sea salt
- 2 tbsps. coconut milk
- 1 tsp. vanilla extract
- 1 cup blueberries

Directions:

1. Set the oven to 400°F. Keep parchment paper on your baking sheet.
2. Add the syrup, flour, salt, and baking powder to a bowl. Combine well by whisking together.
3. Pour the olive oil into a bowl with the dry ingredients.
4. Work the oil into your flour mix.
5. Stir the vanilla extract and coconut milk into the dry ingredients bowl.
6. Fold in the blueberries gently. Your dough should be sticky and thick.
7. Put some flour on your hand then shape the dough into a circle.
8. Take a knife and create triangle slices.
9. Keep them on the baking sheet. Maintain an 8-inch gap.
10. Bake for 25 minutes. Set aside on the baking sheet for cooling once done.

Nutrition:

- **Calories:** 331
- **Carbs:** 27 g
- **Cholesterol:** 0 mg
- **Total Fat:** 23 g
- **Protein:** 4 g
- **Fiber:** 4 g
- **Sugar:** 8 g

CHAPTER 2:

Snacks, Sides, and Appetizers

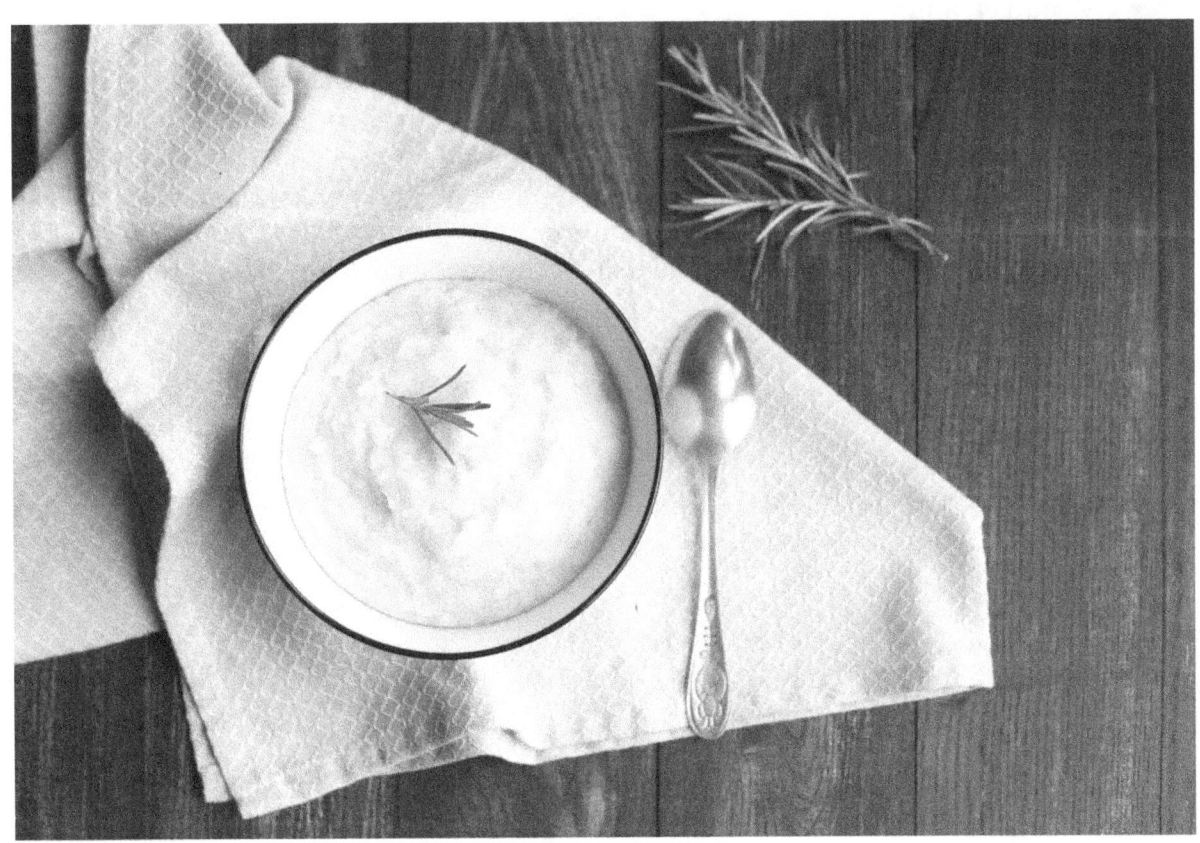

1. Creamy Polenta

Preparation Time: 8 minutes
Cooking Time: 45 minutes
Servings: 4
Ingredients:
- 1 cup polenta
- 1 ½ cup water
- 2 cups chicken stock
- ½ cup cream
- 1/3 cup Parmesan, grated

Directions:
1. Put polenta in the pot.
2. Add water, chicken stock, cream, and Parmesan. Mix up polenta well.
3. Then preheat the oven to 355°F.
4. Cook polenta in the oven for 45 minutes.
5. Mix up the cooked meal with the help of the spoon carefully before serving.

Nutrition:
- **Calories:** 208
- **Fat:** 5.3 g
- **Fiber:** 1 g
- **Carbs:** 32.2 g
- **Protein:** 8 g

2. Mushroom Millet

Preparation Time: 10 minutes
Cooking Time: 15 minutes
Servings: 3
Ingredients:
- ¼ cup mushrooms, sliced
- ¾ cup onion, diced
- 1 tbsp. olive oil
- 1 tsp. salt
- 3 tbsps. milk
- ½ cup millet
- 1 cup water
- 1 tsp. butter

Directions:
1. Pour olive oil into the skillet, then put in the onion.
2. Add mushrooms and roast the vegetables for 10 minutes over medium heat. Stir them from time to time.
3. Meanwhile, pour water into the pan.
4. Add millet and salt.
5. Cook the millet with the closed lid for 15 minutes over medium heat.
6. Then add the cooked mushroom mixture to the millet.
7. Add milk and butter. Mix up the millet well.

Nutrition:
- **Calories:** 198
- **Fat:** 7.7 g
- **Fiber:** 3.5 g
- **Carbs:** 27.9 g
- **Protein:** 4.7 g

3. Roasted Curried Cauliflower

Preparation Time: 5 minutes
Cooking Time: 30 minutes
Servings: 4
Ingredients:
- 1 large head cauliflower, cut into florets
- 1 tsp. curry powder
- 1 ½ tbsp. olive oil
- 1 tsp. cumin seeds
- 1 tsp. mustard seeds
- ¾ tsp. salt

Directions:
1. Preheat your oven to 375°F
2. Grease a baking sheet with cooking spray
3. Take a bowl and place all ingredients
4. Toss to coat well
5. Arrange the vegetable on a baking sheet
6. Roast for 30 minutes
7. Serve and enjoy!

Nutrition:
- **Calories:** 67
- **Fat:** 6 g
- **Carbs:** 4 g
- **Protein:** 2 g

4. Caramelized Pears and Onions

Preparation Time: 5 minutes
Cooking Time: 35 minutes
Servings: 4
Ingredients:
- 2 red onion, cut into wedges
- 2 firm red pears, cored and quartered
- 1 tbsp. olive oil
- Salt and pepper, to taste

Directions:
1. Preheat your oven to 425°F
2. Place the pears and onion on a baking tray
3. Drizzle with olive oil
4. Season with salt and pepper
5. Bake in the oven for 35 minutes
6. Serve and enjoy!

Nutrition:
- **Calories:** 101
- **Fat:** 4 g
- **Carbs:** 17 g
- **Protein:** 1 g

5. Spicy Roasted Brussels Sprouts

Preparation Time: 5 minutes
Cooking Time: 30 minutes
Servings: 4
Ingredients:
- 1 ¼ pound Brussels sprouts, cut into florets
- ½ cup kimchi with juice
- 2 tbsps. olive oil
- Salt and pepper, to taste

Directions:
1. Set the oven to 425°F.
2. Toss the Brussels sprouts with pepper, salt, and oil.
3. Bake in the oven for 25 minutes
4. Remove from oven and mix with kimchi
5. Return to the oven
6. Cook for 5 minutes
7. Serve and enjoy!

Nutrition:
- **Calories:** 135
- **Fat:** 7 g
- **Carbs:** 16 g
- **Protein:** 5 g

6. Apple Sauce Treat

Preparation Time: 10 minutes
Cooking Time: 0 minutes
Servings: 1
Ingredients:
- 1/4 cup low-fat cottage cheese
- 1/4 cup unsweetened applesauce
- 1/2 tsp. cinnamon
- 1 1/2 tsp. toasted slivered almonds

Directions:
1. Mix the cottage cheese and applesauce in a bowl, stirring well.
2. Sprinkle with cinnamon and mix well.
3. Sprinkle the top with almonds, pick up your spoon, and enjoy.

Nutrition:
- **Calories:** 225
- **Protein:** 16.24 g
- **Fat:** 14.17 g
- **Carbs:** 8.54 g

7. Brownies Avocado

Preparation Time: 10 minutes
Cooking Time: 25 minutes
Servings: 6–8
Ingredients:
- 1/2 cup almond meal
- 3/4 cup cocoa powder
- 1 1/2 tsp. instant coffee (with or without caffeine, as you wish)
- 2 tsps. ground cinnamon
- 1/2 tsp. salt
- 2 cups nuts or seeds, chopped
- 1 avocado
- 1 apple, cored and chopped, with the skin on
- 1 cup cooked and diced sweet potato
- 4 tbsps. ground chia seeds
- 1 tsp. vanilla
- 1/2 cup almond butter
- 1/2 cup coconut butter, softened
- 1/4 cup coconut oil
- 2 1/4 cup stevia

Directions:
1. Set the oven to 350°F then line a 9 by 13-inch pan with parchment. Let it overlap the sides to make handles for lifting the brownies out when done.
2. In a bowl, combine the almond meal, cocoa, coffee, cinnamon, salt, and nuts. Whisk and set aside.
3. Bring the rest of the ingredients in a food processor and mix until smooth. Add the ingredients to the bowl and pulse. This combination should be chunky.
4. Pour into pan and bake for at least 25 minutes.
5. Let cool and chill in the refrigerator for two hours before slicing. The baked product will be a little gooey, so refrigerating it makes the brownies easier to cut. The chilled results will be somewhat crumbly.

Nutrition:
- **Calories:** 591
- **Protein:** 11.03 g
- **Fat:** 53.8 g
- **Carbs:** 26.58 g

8. Brussels Sprout Chips

Preparation Time: 10 minutes
Cooking Time: 10 minutes
Servings: 4
Ingredients:
- 2 cups Brussels sprout leaves
- 2 tbsps. ghee
- Kosher salt
- 1 Lemon zest

Directions:
1. Set the oven to 350°F, then cover two cookie sheets with parchment paper.
2. Put the leaves in a big bowl and pour melted ghee over the top, and add salt.
3. Bake for at least 8 to 10 minutes or until the leaves are crispy. If they are soft at all, put them back in the oven.
4. While still hot, sprinkle the lemon zest over the leaves. Serve warm.

Nutrition:
- **Calories:** 42
- **Protein:** 3.13 g
- **Fat:** 1.68 g
- **Carbs:** 4.77 g

9. Cauliflower Snacks

Preparation Time: 10 minutes
Cooking Time: 60 minutes
Servings: 4
Ingredients:
- 1 cauliflower head
- 4 tbsps. extra virgin olive oil
- 1 tsp. salt

Directions:
1. Set the oven to 425°F, then prepare two cookie sheets by lining them with parchment paper.
2. Trim off the cauliflower florets and discard the core. Cut the florets into golf-ball-sized pieces.
3. Place the cauliflower in a bowl and pour olive oil over them and sprinkle with salt. Mix to coat. Spread in a single layer, not touching.
4. Roast about 1 hour, turning the cauliflower three to four times until golden brown. Serve warm.

Nutrition:
- **Calories:** 91
- **Protein:** 2.93 g
- **Fat:** 7.7 g
- **Carbs:** 3.29 g

10. Ginger Flour Banana Ginger Bars

Preparation Time: 10 minutes
Cooking Time: 40 minutes
Servings: 4–6
Ingredients:
- 1 cup coconut flour
- 1 ½ tbsp. grated ginger
- 2 large ripe bananas
- 1 tsp. baking soda
- 1/3 cup melted butter
- 2 tsp. cinnamon
- 2 tsp. apple cider vinegar
- 1/3 cup honey or maple syrup
- 1 tsp. ground cardamom
- 6 medium while eggs

Directions:
1. Preheat the oven to 350°F.
2. Line a glass baking dish with parchment paper. If you don't have any paper, just grease the pan.
3. Put all the ingredients except the baking soda and apple cider vinegar through a food processor and blend until it's all mixed up.
4. Now add the last two ingredients and blitz once before pouring the mix into the glass dish.
5. Bake up to a toothpick inserted into the center comes out clean. This usually takes 40 minutes.

Nutrition:
- **Calories:** 1407
- **Protein:** 42.18 g
- **Fat:** 100.26 g
- **Carbs:** 88.33 g

11. Tangy Turmeric Flavored Florets

Preparation Time: 10 minutes
Cooking Time: 55 minutes
Servings: 1

Ingredients:
- 1 cauliflower head, chopped into florets
- 1 tbsp. olive oil
- 1 tbsp. turmeric
- A pinch of cumin
- A dash of salt

Directions:
1. Set the oven to 400°F.
2. Put all the ingredients in a baking pan. Mix well until thoroughly combined.
3. Cover the pan with foil. Roast for 40 minutes. Remove the foil cover and roast additionally for 15 minutes.

Nutrition:
- **Calories:** 90
- **Fat:** 3 g
- **Protein:** 4.5 g
- **Sodium:** 87 mg
- **Total carbs:** 16.2 g
- **Dietary Fiber:** 5 g
- **Net Carbs:** 11.2 g

12. Cool Garbanzo and Spinach Beans

Preparation Time: 5-10 minutes
Cooking Time: 5 minutes
Servings: 4
Ingredients:
- 12 oz. garbanzo beans
- 1 tbsp. olive oil
- ½ onion, diced
- ½ tsp. cumin
- 10 oz. spinach, chopped

Directions:
1. Take a skillet and add olive oil.
2. Place it over medium-low heat.
3. Add onions, garbanzo and cook for 5 minutes.
4. Stir in cumin, garbanzo beans, spinach, and season with sunflower seeds.
5. Use a spoon to smash gently.
6. Cook thoroughly.
7. Serve and enjoy!

Nutrition:
- **Calories:** 90
- **Fat:** 4 g
- **Carbs:** 11 g
- **Protein:** 4 g

13. Onion and Orange Healthy Salad

Preparation Time: 10 minutes
Cooking Time: 0 minutes
Servings: 3
Ingredients:
- 6 large oranges
- 3 tbsps. red wine vinegar
- 6 tbsps. olive oil
- 1 tsp. dried oregano
- 1 red onion, thinly sliced
- 1 cup olive oil
- ¼ cup fresh chives, chopped
- Ground black pepper

Directions:
1. Peel the orange and cut each of them into 4–5 crosswise slices.
2. Transfer the oranges to a shallow dish.
3. Drizzle vinegar, olive oil, and sprinkle oregano. Toss.
4. Chill for 30 minutes.
5. Arrange sliced onion and black olives on top.
6. Decorate with an additional sprinkle of chives and a fresh grind of pepper.
7. Serve and enjoy!

Nutrition:
- **Calories:** 120
- **Fat:** 6 g
- **Carbs:** 20 g
- **Protein:** 2 g

14. Oven Crisp Sweet Potato

Preparation Time: 10 minutes
Cooking Time: 20 minutes
Servings: 2
Ingredients:
- 1 medium-sized sweet potato, raw
- 1 tsp. sugar
- 1 tsp. coconut oil

Directions:
1. Preheat the oven to 160°C.
2. Using a mandolin slicer or a peeler, slice the sweet potato into thin chips or strips. Wash and pat dry.
3. Drizzle the coconut oil over the potatoes. Toss until all chips are coated.
4. Arrange in an oven baking sheet. Bake for 10 minutes. Check the crispiness. If it is not that crispy enough, bake for another 5 or 10 minutes or until the chips attain the crispiness desired.
5. Take out the crispy sweet potatoes. Sprinkle with sugar and serve.

Nutrition:
- **Calories:** 123
- **Protein:** 4.23 g
- **Fat:** 5.39 g
- **Carbs:** 14.63 g

15. Olive and Tomato Balls

Preparation Time: 10 minutes
Cooking Time: 35 minutes
Servings: 5
Ingredients:

- 5 tbsps. parmesan cheese, grated
- ¼ tsp. salt
- black pepper (as desired)
- 2 garlic cloves, crushed
- 4 kalamata olives, pitted
- 4 pcs. sun-dried tomatoes, drained
- 2 tbsps. oregano, chopped
- 2 tbsps. thyme, chopped
- 2 tbsps. basil, chopped
- ¼ cup coconut oil
- ½ cup cream cheese

Directions:

1. Chop the coconut oil, add it to a small mixing bowl with the cream cheese, and leave them to soften for about 30 minutes. Mash together and mix well to combine.
2. Add in the Kalamata olives and sun-dried tomatoes and mix well before adding in the herbs and seasonings. Combine thoroughly before placing the mixing bowl in the refrigerator to allow the results to solidify.
3. Once it has solidified, form the mixture into a total of 5 balls using an ice cream scoop. Roll each of the finished balls into the parmesan cheese before plating.
4. Store the extra's in the fridge in an air-tight container for up to 7 days.

Nutrition:

- **Calories:** 212
- **Protein:** 4.77 g
- **Fat:** 20.75 g
- **Carbs:** 3.13 g

16. Stir-Fried Almond and Spinach

Preparation Time: 10 minutes
Cooking Time: 15 minutes
Servings: 2
Ingredients:
- 34 pounds spinach
- 3 tbsps. almonds
- Salt to taste
- 1 tbsp. coconut oil

Directions:
1. Put oil into a large pot and place it on high heat.
2. Add spinach and let it cook, stirring frequently.
3. Once the spinach is cooked and tender, season with salt and stir.
4. Add almonds and enjoy!

Nutrition:
- **Calories:** 150
- **Fat:** 12 g
- **Carbs:** 10 g
- **Protein:** 8 g

17. Cilantro and Avocado Platter

Preparation Time: 10 minutes
Cooking Time: 0 minutes
Servings: 6
Ingredients:
- 2 avocados, peeled, pitted and diced
- 1 sweet onion, chopped
- 1 green bell pepper, chopped
- 1 large ripe tomato, chopped
- ¼ cup fresh cilantro, chopped
- ½ lime, juiced
- Salt and pepper as needed

Directions:
1. Take a medium-sized bowl and add onion, bell pepper, tomato, avocados, lime, and cilantro.
2. Mix well and give it a toss.
3. Season with salt, and pepper according to your taste.
4. Serve and enjoy!

Nutrition:
- **Calories:** 126
- **Fat:** 10 g
- **Carbs:** 10 g
- **Protein:** 2 g

18. Spicy Barley

Preparation Time: 7 minutes
Cooking Time: 42 minutes
Servings: 5

Ingredients:
- 1 cup barley
- 3 cups chicken stock
- ½ tsp. cayenne pepper
- 1 tsp. salt
- ½ tsp. chili pepper
- ½ tsp. ground black pepper
- 1 tsp. butter
- 1 tsp. olive oil

Directions:
1. Place barley and olive oil in the pan.
2. Roast barley on high heat for 1 minute. Stir it well.
3. Then add salt, chili pepper, ground black pepper, cayenne pepper, and butter.
4. Add chicken stock.
5. Close the lid and cook barley for 40 minutes over medium-low heat.

Nutrition:
- **Calories:** 152
- **Fat:** 2.9 g
- **Fiber:** 6.5 g
- **Carbs:** 27.8 g
- **Protein:** 5.1 g

19. Tender Farro

Preparation Time: 8 minutes
Cooking Time: 40 minutes
Servings: 4
Ingredients:
- 1 cup farro
- 3 cups beef broth
- 1 tsp. salt
- 1 tbsp. almond butter
- 1 tbsp. dried dill

Directions:
1. Place the farro in the pan.
2. Add beef broth, dried dill, and salt.
3. Close the lid and place the mixture to boil.
4. Then boil it for 35 minutes over medium-low heat.
5. When the time is done, open the lid and add almond butter.
6. Mix up the cooked the farro well.

Nutrition:
- **Calories:** 95
- **Fat:** 3.3 g
- **Fiber:** 1.3 g
- **Carbs:** 10.1 g
- **Protein:** 6.4 g

20. Wheatberry Salad

Preparation Time: 10 minutes
Cooking Time: 50 minutes
Servings: 2
Ingredients:
- ¼ cup wheat berries
- 1 cup water
- 1 tsp. salt
- 2 tbsps. walnuts, chopped
- 1 tbsp. chives, chopped
- ¼ cup fresh parsley, chopped
- 2 oz. pomegranate seeds
- 1 tbsp. canola oil
- 1 tsp. chili flakes

Directions:
1. Place wheat berries and water in the pan.
2. Add salt and simmer the ingredients for 50 minutes over medium heat.
3. Meanwhile, mix up together walnuts, chives, parsley, pomegranate seeds, and chili flakes.
4. When the wheat berry is cooked, transfer it to the walnut mixture.
5. Add canola oil and mix up the salad well.

Nutrition:
- **Calories:** 160
- **Fat:** 11.8 g
- **Fiber:** 1.2 g
- **Carbs:** 12 g
- **Protein:** 3.4 g

CHAPTER 3:

Lunch

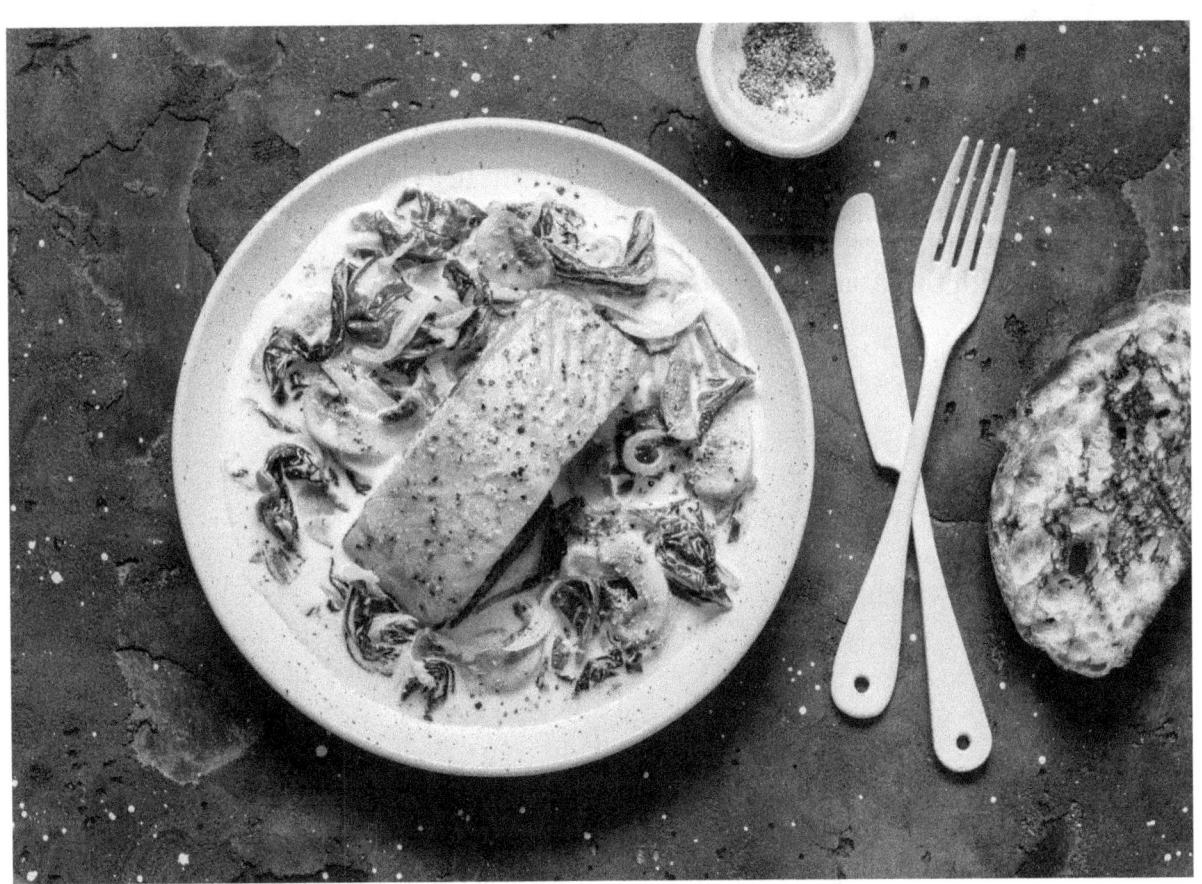

1. Pan-Seared Scallops with Lemon-Ginger Vinaigrette

Preparation Time: 10 minutes
Cooking Time: 7 minutes
Servings: 4
Ingredients:
- 2 tbsps. extra virgin olive oil
- 1 ½ pound sea scallop
- ½ tsp. sea salt
- ⅛ tsp. freshly ground black pepper
- ¼ cup lemon ginger vinaigrette

Directions:
1. In a big nonstick skillet at medium-high heat, heat the olive oil until it shimmers.
2. Season the scallops with pepper and salt and add them to the skillet. Cook for at least 3 minutes per side until just opaque.
3. Serve with the vinaigrette spooned over the top.

Nutrition:
- **Calories:** 280
- **Total Fat:** 16
- **Total carbs:** 5 g
- **Sugar:** 1 g
- **Fiber:** 0 g
- **Protein:** 29 g
- **Sodium:** 508 mg

2. Manhattan-Style Salmon Chowder

Preparation Time: 10 minutes
Cooking Time: 15 minutes
Servings: 4
Ingredients:

- ¼ cup extra virgin olive oil
- 1 red bell pepper, chopped
- 1 pound skinless salmon. pin bones removed, chopped into ½ inch
- 2 (28 oz.) cans crushed tomatoes, 1 drained, 1 undrained
- 6 cups no-salt-added chicken broth
- 2 cups diced (1/2 inch) sweet potato
- 1 tsp. onion powder
- ½ tsp. sea salt
- ¼ tsp. freshly ground black pepper

Directions:

Add the red bell pepper and salmon. Cook for at least 5 minutes, occasionally stirring, until the fish is opaque and the bell pepper is soft.

Stir in the tomatoes, chicken broth, sweet potatoes, onion powder, salt, and pepper. Place to a simmer, then lower the heat to medium. Cook for at least 10 minutes, occasionally stirring, until the sweet potatoes are soft.

Nutrition:

- **Calories:** 570
- **Total Fat:** 42
- **Total carbs:** 55 g
- **Sugar:** 24 g
- **Fiber:** 16 g
- **Protein:** 41 g
- **Sodium:** 1,249 mg

3. Sesame-Tuna Skewers

Preparation Time: 10 minutes
Cooking Time: 15 minutes
Servings: 6
Ingredients:
- 6 oz. cubed thick tuna steaks
- Cooking spray
- ¼ tsp. ground black pepper.
- ¾ cup sesame seeds
- 1 tsp. salt
- ½ tsp. ground ginger.
- 2 tbsps. toasted sesame oil

Directions:
1. Preheat the oven to about 400°F.
2. Coat a rimmed baking tray with cooking spray.
3. Soak twelve wooden skewers in water
4. In a small mixing bowl, combine pepper, ground ginger, salt, and sesame seeds.
5. In another bowl, toss the tuna with sesame oil.
6. Press the oiled cubes into a sesame seed mixture and put the cubes on each skewer.
7. Put the skewers on a readily prepared baking tray and put the tray into the preheated oven.
8. Bake for 12 minutes and turn once.
9. Serve and enjoy.

Nutrition:
- **Calories:** 196
- **Protein:** 14.47 g
- **Fat:** 15.01 g
- **Carbs:** 2.48 g

4. Trout with Chard

Preparation Time: 10 minutes
Cooking Time: 15 minutes
Servings: 4
Ingredients:
- ½ cup vegetable broth
- 2 bunches of sliced chard
- 4 boneless trout fillets
- Salt
- 1 tbsp. extra virgin olive oil
- 2 minced garlic cloves
- ¼ cup golden raisins
- Ground black pepper
- 1 chopped onion
- 1 tbsp. apple cider vinegar

Directions:
1. Preheat the oven to about 375°F.
2. Add seasonings to the trout
3. Add olive oil in a pan, then heat.
4. Add garlic and onion, then sauté for 3 minutes.
5. Add chard to sauté for 2 more minutes.
6. Add broth, raisins, and cedar vinegar to the pan.
7. Layer a topping of trout fillets
8. Cover the pan and put it in the preheated oven for 10 minutes.
9. Serve and enjoy.

Nutrition:
- **Calories:** 284
- **Protein:** 2.07 g
- **Fat:** 30.32 g
- **Carbs:** 3.49 g

5. Seafood Noodles

Preparation Time: 10 minutes
Cooking Time: 20 minutes
Servings: 2
Ingredients:
- Braised olive oil
- 4 garlic cloves, minced
- 300 g clean squid cut into rings
- 200 g mussel without shell
- 200 g shell-less volley
- 10 clean prawns
- 150 g dried tomatoes
- Salt to taste
- black pepper to taste
- 500 g pre-cooked noodles
- ½ pack watercress
- ½ Lemon Juice
- parsley to taste

Directions:
1. In olive oil, sauté the garlic and add the squid, the mussel, the shrimp, and the shrimp.
2. Put the dried tomatoes and season with salt and pepper.
3. Add the noodles, watercress, season with lemon juice and parsley.

Nutrition:
- **Calories:** 2049
- **Protein:** 56.21 g
- **Fat:** 143.36 g
- **Carbs:** 139.98 g

6. Spicy Pulled Chicken Wraps

Preparation Time: 15 minutes
Cooking Time: 6 to 8 hours
Servings: 4
Ingredients:
- 1 romaine lettuce head
- 1 ½ tsp. ground cumin
- 1 ½ cup low-fat, low-sodium chicken broth
- 1 tsp. paprika
- 1 tsp. garlic powder
- 1 lb. skinless, deboned chicken breasts
- 2 tsps. chili powder

Directions:
1. In a slow cooker, put all the ingredients except lettuce and gently stir to combine.
2. Set the slow cooker on low.
3. Cover and cook for about 6–8 hours.
4. Uncover the slow cooker and transfer the breasts to a large plate.
5. With a fork, shred the breasts.
6. Serve the shredded beef over lettuce leaves.

Nutrition:
- **Calories:** 150
- **Fat:** 3.4 g
- **Carbs:** 12 g
- **Protein:** 14 g
- **Sugars:** 7 g
- **Sodium:** 900 mg

7. Apricot Chicken Wings

Preparation Time: 15 minutes
Cooking Time: 45–60 minutes
Servings: 3–4
Ingredients:
- 1 medium jar apricot preserve
- 1 package Lipton® onion dry soup mix
- 1 medium bottle Russian dressing
- 2 lbs. chicken wings

Directions:
1. Preheat the oven to 350°F.
2. Rinse and pat dry the chicken wings.
3. Bring the chicken wings on a baking pan, single layer.
4. Bake for 45–60 minutes, turning halfway.
5. In a medium bowl, combine the Lipton® soup mix, apricot preserve, and Russian dressing.
6. Once the wings are cooked, toss with the sauce, until the pieces are coated.
7. Serve immediately with a side dish.

Nutrition:
- **Calories:** 162
- **Fat:** 17 g
- **Carbs:** 76 g
- **Protein:** 13 g
- **Sugars:** 24 g
- **Sodium:** 700 mg

8. Champion Chicken Pockets

Preparation Time: 5 minutes
Cooking Time: 0 minutes
Servings: 4
Ingredients:
- ½ cup chopped broccoli
- 2 halved whole wheat pita bread rounds
- ¼ cup bottled reduced-fat ranch salad dressing
- ¼ cup chopped pecans or walnuts
- 1 ½ cup chopped cooked chicken
- ¼ cup plain low-fat yogurt
- ¼ cup shredded carrot

Directions:
1. In a bowl, put together yogurt and ranch salad dressing, then mix.
2. In a medium bowl, combine chicken, broccoli, carrot, and, if desired, nuts. Pour yogurt mixture over chicken; toss to coat.
3. Spoon chicken mixture into pita halves.

Nutrition:
- **Calories:** 384
- **Fat:** 11.4 g
- **Carbs:** 7.4 g
- **Protein:** 59.3 g
- **Sugars:** 1.3 g
- **Sodium:** 368.7 mg

9. Chicken-Bell Pepper Sauté

Preparation Time: 10 minutes
Cooking Time: 30 minutes
Servings: 6
Ingredients:
- 1 tbsp. olive oil
- 1 sliced large yellow bell pepper
- 1 sliced large red bell pepper
- 3 cup onion sliced crosswise
- 6 4-oz skinless, boneless chicken breast halves
- Cooking spray
- 20 Kalamata olives
- ¼ tsp. Freshly ground black pepper
- ½ tsp. salt
- 2 tbsps. finely chopped fresh flat-leaf parsley
- 2 1/3 cup coarsely chopped tomato
- 1 tsp. chopped fresh oregano

Directions:
1. Adjust your heat to medium-high and set non-stick frying in place. Heat the oil. Sauté the onions for 8 minutes once the oil is hot.
2. Add bell pepper and sauté for 10 more minutes.
3. Add tomato, salt, and black pepper to cook for about 7 minutes until the tomato juice has evaporated.
4. Add parsley, oregano, and olives to cook for 2 minutes until heated. Set into a bowl and keep warm.
5. Using a paper towel, wipe the pan and grease with cooking spray. Set back to heat and add chicken breasts. Cook for 3 more minutes on each of the sides. You can opt to cook the chicken in batches
6. When cooking the last batch, add back the previous batch of chicken and onion-bell pepper mixture, then cook for a minute as you toss.
7. Serve warm and enjoy.

Nutrition:
- **Calories:** 223
- **Protein:** 28.13 g
- **Fat:** 7.82 g
- **Carbs:** 9.5 g

10. Curried Beef Meatballs

Preparation Time: 20 minutes
Cooking Time: 22 minutes
Servings: 6
Ingredients:
For Meatballs:
- 1 pound lean ground beef
- 2 organic eggs, beaten
- 3 tbsps. red onion, minced
- ¼ cup fresh basil leaves, chopped
- 1 (1-inch) fresh ginger piece, chopped finely
- 4 garlic cloves, chopped finely
- 3 Thai birds-eye chilies, minced
- 1 tsp. coconut sugar
- 1 tbsp. red curry paste
- Salt, to taste
- 1 tbsp. fish sauce
- 2 tbsps. coconut oil

For Curry:
- 1 red onion, chopped - Salt, to taste
- 4 garlic cloves, minced
- 1 (1-inch) fresh ginger piece, minced
- 2 Thai birds-eye chilies, minced
- 2 tbsps. red curry paste - 1 (14 oz.) coconut milk
- Salt, to taste
- Freshly ground black pepper, to taste
- Lime wedges (as desired)

Directions:
1. For meatballs in a big bowl, put all the ingredients except oil and mix until well combined. Make small balls from the mixture.
2. In a big skillet, melt coconut oil on medium heat.
3. Add meatballs and cook for about 3–5 minutes or till golden brown on all sides.
4. Transfer the meatballs right into a bowl. In the same skillet, add onion and a pinch of salt and sauté for around 5 minutes.
5. Add garlic, ginger, and chilies, and sauté for about 1 minute.
6. Add curry paste and sauté for around 1 minute. Add coconut milk and meatballs and convey to some gentle simmer. Reduce the warmth to low and simmer, covered for around 10 minutes. Serve using the topping of lime wedges.

Nutrition:
- **Calories:** 444 **Fat:** 15 g **Carbs:** 20 g **Fiber:** 2 g **Protein:** 37 g

11. Beef Meatballs in Tomato Gravy

Preparation Time: 20 minutes
Cooking Time: 37 minutes
Servings: 4
Ingredients:
For Meatballs:
- 1 pound lean ground beef
- 1 organic egg, beaten
- 1 tbsp. fresh ginger, minced
- 1 garlic oil, minced
- 2 tbsps. fresh cilantro, chopped finely
- 2 tbsps. tomato paste - 1/3 cup almond meal
- 1 tbsp. ground cumin - A pinch of ground cinnamon
- Salt, to taste - Freshly ground black pepper, to taste
- ¼ cup coconut oil

For Tomato Gravy:
- 2 tbsps. coconut oil - ½ small onion, chopped
- 2 garlic cloves, chopped
- 1 tsp. fresh lemon zest, grated finely
- 2 cups tomatoes, chopped finely - A pinch of ground cinnamon
- 1 tsp. red pepper flakes, crushed
- ¾ cup chicken broth - Salt, to taste
- Freshly ground black pepper, to taste
- ¼ cup fresh parsley, chopped

Directions:
1. For meatballs in a sizable bowl, add all ingredients except oil and mix until well combined. Make about 1-inch sized balls from the mixture.
2. In a substantial skillet, melt coconut oil into medium heat.
3. Add meatballs and cook for approximately 3–5 minutes or till golden brown on all sides. Transfer the meatballs into a bowl.
4. For gravy in a big pan, melt coconut oil into medium heat.
5. Add onion and garlic and sauté for approximately 4 minutes.
6. Add lemon zest and sauté for approximately 1 minute.
7. Add tomatoes, cinnamon, red pepper flakes, and broth and simmer for approximately 7 minutes.
8. Stir in salt, black pepper, and meatballs and reduce the warmth to medium-low.
9. Simmer for approximately twenty minutes.
10. Serve hot with all the garnishing of parsley.

Nutrition:
- **Calories:** 404 **Fat:** 11 g **Carbs:** 27 g **Fiber:** 4 g **Protein:** 38 g

12. Pork with Lemongrass

Preparation Time: 10 minutes
Cooking Time: 30 minutes
Servings: 4
Ingredients:
- 4 pork chops
- 2 tbsps. olive oil
- 2 spring onions, chopped
- A pinch of salt and black pepper
- ½ cup vegetable stock
- 1 stalk lemongrass, chopped
- 2 tbsps. coconut aminos
- 2 tbsps. cilantro, chopped

Directions:
1. Warm a pan with the oil on medium-high heat, add the spring onions, and the meat, and brown for 5 minutes.
2. Add the rest of the ingredients, toss, and cook everything over medium heat for 25 minutes.
3. Divide the mix between plates and serve.

Nutrition:
- **Calories:** 290
- **Fat:** 4 g
- **Fiber:** 6 g
- **Carbs:** 8 g
- **Protein:** 14 g

13. Pork with Olives

Preparation Time: 10 minutes
Cooking Time: 40 minutes
Servings: 4
Ingredients:
- 1 yellow onion, chopped
- 4 pork chops
- 2 tbsps. olive oil
- 1 tbsp. sweet paprika
- 2 tbsps. balsamic vinegar
- ¼ cup Kalamata olives, pitted and chopped
- 1 tbsp. cilantro, chopped
- A pinch of Sea Salt
- A pinch of black pepper

Directions:
1. Warm a pan with the oil on medium heat; add the onion and sauté for 5 minutes.
2. Add the meat and brown for a further 5 minutes.
3. Put the rest of the ingredients, toss, cook over medium heat for 30 minutes, divide between plates and serve.

Nutrition:
- **Calories:** 280
- **Fat:** 11 g
- **Fiber:** 6 g
- **Carbs:** 10 g
- **Protein:** 21 g

14. Avocado-Orange Grilled Chicken

Preparation Time: 10 minutes
Cooking Time: 12 minutes
Servings: 4
Ingredients:

- 1 cup low-fat yogurt
- Salt
- 4 pieces of 4–6oz boneless, skinless chicken breasts
- 2 tbsps. chopped cilantro
- 1 tbsp. honey
- 1 thinly sliced small red onion
- ¼ cup fresh lime juice
- 1 deseeded avocado, peeled and chopped
- 2 peeled and sectioned oranges
- Pepper
- ¼ cup minced red onion

Directions:

1. Set up a large mixing bowl and mix yogurt, minced red onion, cilantro, and honey.
2. Add chicken into the mixture and marinate for half an hour.
3. Grease grate and preheat the grill to medium-high heat.
4. Set the chicken aside and add seasonings.
5. Grill for 6 minutes on each side.
6. Set the avocado in a bowl.
7. Add lime juice and toss avocado to coat well.
8. Add oranges, thinly sliced onions, and cilantro into the bowl with avocado and combine well.
9. Serve avocado dressing alongside grilled chicken.
10. Enjoy.

Nutrition:

- **Calories:** 216
- **Protein:** 8.83 g
- **Fat:** 11.48 g
- **Carbs:** 21.86 g

15. Honey Chicken Tagine

Preparation Time: 60 minutes
Cooking Time: 25 minutes
Servings: 12
Ingredients:
- 1 tbsp. extra virgin olive oil
- 1 tsp. ground coriander
- 1 tbsp. Minced fresh ginger
- ½ tsp. ground pepper
- 2 thinly sliced onions
- 12 oz. seeded and roughly chopped kumquats
- 14 oz. vegetable broth
- 1/8 tsp. Ground cloves
- ½ tsp. salt
- 1 ½ tbsps. honey
- 1 tsp. ground cumin
- 2 lbs. boneless, skinless chicken thighs
- 4 slivered garlic cloves
- 15 oz. rinsed chickpeas
- ¾ tsp. ground cinnamon

Directions:
1. Preheat the oven to about 375°F.
2. Put a heatproof casserole on medium heat and heat the oil.
3. Add onions to sauté for 4 minutes.
4. Add garlic and ginger to sauté for 1 minute.
5. Add coriander, cumin, cloves, salt, pepper, and cloves seasonings. Sauté for a minute.
6. Add kumquats, broth, chickpeas, and honey, then bring to a boil before turning off the heat.
7. Set the casserole in the oven while covered. Bake for 15 minutes as you stir at a 15-minute interval.
8. Serve and enjoy.

Nutrition:
- **Calories:** 586
- **Protein:** 15.5 g
- **Fat:** 40.82 g
- **Carbs:** 43.56 g

16. Potato Dumpling with Shrimp

Preparation Time: 15 minutes
Cooking Time: 50 minutes
Servings: 6–8
Ingredients:
- 500 g pink potatoes
- 1 egg
- Salt to taste
- 1 tbsp chopped parsley
- 2 tbsps. flour + flour for handling and breading
- 10 units of clean giant tailed shrimp
- black pepper to taste
- ½ packet of chopped cilantro
- 3 tbsps. palm oil
- 4 lemon juice
- Frying oil

Directions:
1. Put the potato to cook for 40 minutes.
2. When very tender, remove from heat, let cool, and mashed potatoes already peeled.
3. Add the egg and mix well, season with salt and parsley, and add the flour. Set aside in the fridge for 2 hours.
4. Make small transverse cuts on the belly of the shrimp, without cutting to the end. Season the shrimp with black pepper, salt chopped coriander, palm oil, and lemon juice. Leave marinating for 15 minutes.
5. Take a portion of the potato flour dough in your hands and shape around a shrimp, leaving the tail out.
6. Rinse flour again and fry in hot oil until golden.

Nutrition:
- **Calories:** 159
- **Protein:** 6.95 g
- **Fat:** 8.42 g
- **Carbs:** 14.48 g

17. Shrimp Rissoles

Preparation Time: 10 minutes
Cooking Time: 30 minutes
Servings: 4
Ingredients:
- 1 tbsp. olive oil
- ½ diced onion
- 400 g shrimp
- 2 tbsp. tomato extract
- ½ packet chopped parsley
- Salt to taste
- 250 ml of water
- 250 ml milk
- 50 g butter
- 3 cups flour
- 100 g curd
- 3 beaten eggs
- Breadcrumbs for breading

Directions:
1. Sauté with olive oil, onion, and shrimp.
2. Add tomato extract, parsley, and salt. Reserve.
3. In a pan, bring to medium heat water, milk and butter.
4. When the butter has melted, add 2 cups of wheat flour at a time and stir until the dough begins to unglue from the bottom of the pan. Set aside until warm.
5. When the dough is warm, knead, adding the remaining flour until it is smooth and elastic.
6. Roll the dough into a floured surface.
7. The format in circular portions.
8. Stuff with the shrimp and arrange a spoonful of curd. Close by tightening the ends.
9. Dip into beaten egg, breadcrumbs, and fry in hot oil until golden brown.

Nutrition:
- **Calories:** 736
- **Protein:** 42.45 g
- **Fat:** 26.71 g
- **Carbs:** 78.58 g

18. Sole with Vegetables

Preparation Time: 10 minutes
Cooking Time: 15 minutes
Servings: 4
Ingredients:
- 4 tsp. divided extra virgin olive oil
- 1 thinly sliced and divided carrot
- Salt
- 1 lemon wedges (as desired)
- ½ cup divided vegetable broth
- 5 oz. sole fillets
- 2 sliced and thinly divided shallots
- Ground black pepper
- 2 tbsps. divided snipped fresh chives
- 1 thinly sliced and divided zucchini

Directions:
1. Preheat the oven to about 425°F.
2. Separate the aluminum foil into medium-sized pieces
3. Put a fillet on one half of the aluminum foil piece and add seasonings
4. Add shallots, zucchini, and ¼ each of the carrots on top of the fillet. Sprinkle with 1 ½ tsp. of chives
5. Drizzle 2 tbsps. of broth and a tbsp. of olive oil over the fish and vegetables
6. Seal to make a packet and put the packet on a large baking tray.
7. Repeat for the rest of the ingredients and make more packets
8. Put the sheet in a preheated oven and bake the packets for 15 minutes
9. Peel back the foil and put the contents with the liquid onto a serving plate.
10. Garnish with lemon wedges before serving.
11. Enjoy.

Nutrition:
- **Calories:** 130
- **Protein:** 9.94 g
- **Fat:** 7.96 g
- **Carbs:** 4.92 g

19. Roasted Salmon and Asparagus

Preparation Time: 5 minutes
Cooking Time: 15 minutes
Servings: 4
Ingredients:
- 1 pound asparagus spears, trimmed
- 2 tbsps. extra virgin olive oil
- 1 tsp. sea salt, divide
- 1 ½ pound salmon, cut into 4 fillets
- ⅛ tsp. freshly ground cracked black pepper
- 1 lemon, zest, and slice

Directions:
1. Preheat the oven to 425°F.
2. Stir the asparagus with the olive oil, then put ½ tsp. of the salt. Place in a single layer in the bottom of a roasting pan.
3. Season the salmon with the pepper and the remaining ½ tsp. of salt. Put skin-side down on top of the asparagus.
4. Sprinkle the salmon and asparagus with the lemon zest and place the lemon slices over the fish.
5. Roast at the oven for at least 12 to 15 minutes until the flesh is opaque.

Nutrition:
- **Calories:** 308
- **Total Fat:** 18 g
- **Total carbs:** 5 g
- **Sugar:** 2 g
- **Fiber:** 2 g
- **Protein:** 36 g
- **Sodium:** 545 mg

20. Citrus Salmon on a Bed of Greens

Preparation Time: 10 minutes
Cooking Time: 19 minutes
Servings: 4
Ingredients:

- ¼ cup extra virgin olive oil, divided
- 1 ½ pound salmon
- 1 tsp. sea salt, divided
- ½ tsp. freshly ground black pepper, divided
- 1 lemon zest
- 6 cups swiss chard, stemmed and chopped
- 3 garlic cloves, chopped
- 2 lemon juice

Directions:

1. In a big nonstick skillet at medium-high heat, heat 2 tbsps. of olive oil until it shimmers.
2. Season the salmon with ½ tsp. of the salt, ¼ tsp. of the pepper, and the lemon zest. Put the salmon in the skillet, skin-side up, and cook for about 7 minutes until the flesh is opaque. Flip the salmon and cook for at least 3 to 4 minutes to crisp the skin. Set aside on a plate, cover using aluminum foil.
3. Put back the skillet to the heat, add the remaining 2 tbsps. of olive oil, and heat it until it shimmers.
4. Add the Swiss chard. Cook for about 7 minutes, occasionally stirring, until soft.
5. Add the garlic. Cook for 30 seconds, stirring constantly.
6. Sprinkle in the lemon juice, the remaining ½ tsp. of salt, and the remaining ¼ tsp. of pepper. Cook for 2 minutes.
7. Serve the salmon on the Swiss chard.

Nutrition:

- **Calories:** 363
- **Total Fat:** 25
- **Total carbs:** 3 g
- **Sugar:** 1 g
- **Fiber:** 1 g
- **Protein:** 34 g
- **Sodium:** 662 mg

21. Orange and Maple-Glazed Salmon

Preparation Time: 15 minutes
Cooking Time: 15 minutes
Servings: 4
Ingredients:
- 2 orange juice
- 1 orange zest
- ¼ cup pure maple syrup
- 2 tbsp. low sodium soy sauce
- 1 tsp. garlic powder
- 4 4–6 oz. salmon fillet, pin bones removed

Directions:
1. Preheat the oven to 400°F.
2. In a small, shallow dish, whisk the orange juice and zest, maple syrup, soy sauce, and garlic powder.
3. Put the salmon pieces, flesh-side down, into the dish. Let it marinate for 10 minutes.
4. Transfer the salmon, skin-side up, to a rimmed baking sheet, and bake for about 15 minutes until the flesh is opaque.

Nutrition:
- **Calories:** 297
- **Total Fat:** 11
- **Total carbs:** 18 g
- **Sugar:** 15 g
- **Fiber:** 1 g
- **Protein:** 34 g
- **Sodium:** 528 mg

CHAPTER 4:

Dinner

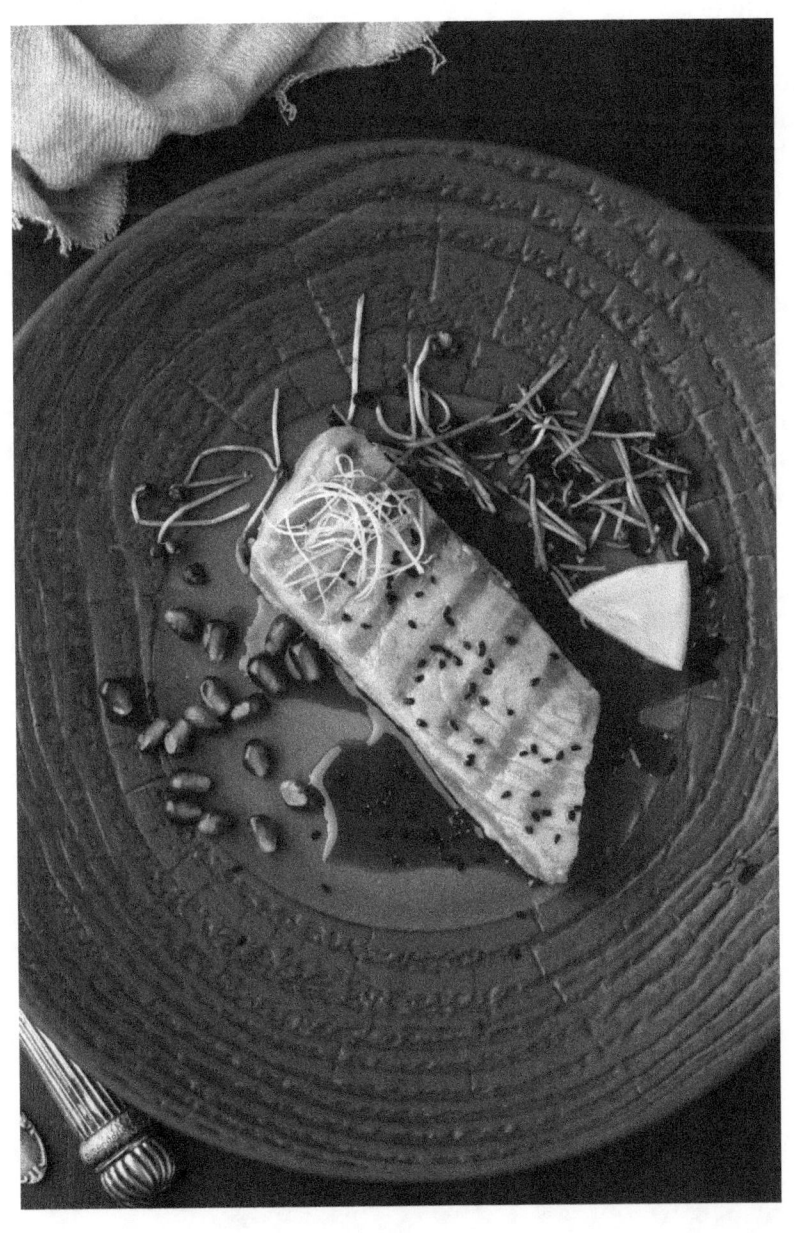

1. Lemony Mussels

Preparation Time: 5 minutes
Cooking Time: 5 minutes
Servings: 4
Ingredients:
- 1 tbsp. extra virgin olive oil
- 2 minced garlic cloves
- 2 lbs. scrubbed mussels
- 1 lemon juice

Directions:
1. Put some water in a pot, add mussels, bring with a boil over medium heat, cook for 5 minutes, discard unopened mussels and transfer them with a bowl.
2. In another bowl, mix the oil with garlic and freshly squeezed lemon juice, whisk well, and add over the mussels, toss and serve.
3. Enjoy!

Nutrition:
- **Calories:** 140
- **Fat:** 4 g
- **Carbs:** 8 g
- **Protein:** 8 g
- **Sugars:** 4 g
- **Sodium:** 600 mg

2. Hot Tuna Steak

Preparation Time: 10 minutes
Cooking Time: 25 minutes
Servings: 6
Ingredients:
- 2 tbsps. fresh lemon juice
- Pepper
- roasted orange garlic mayonnaise
- ¼ cup whole black peppercorns
- 6 sliced tuna steaks
- 2 tbsps. extra virgin olive oil
- Salt

Directions:
1. Bring the tuna in a bowl to fit. Put the oil, lemon juice, salt, and pepper. Turn the tuna to coat well in the marinade.
2. Rest for at least 15 to 20 minutes, turning once.
3. Put the peppercorns in a double thickness of plastic bags. Tap the peppercorns with a heavy saucepan or small mallet to crush them coarsely. Put on a large plate.
4. Once ready to cook the tuna, dip the edges into the crushed peppercorns. Heat a nonstick skillet over medium heat. Sear the tuna steaks in batches if necessary, for 4 minutes per side for medium-rare fish, adding 2 to 3 tbsps. of the marinade to the skillet if necessary, to prevent sticking.
5. Serve dolloped with roasted orange garlic mayonnaise.

Nutrition:
- **Calories:** 124
- **Fat:** 0.4 g
- **Carbs:** 0.6 g
- **Protein:** 28 g
- **Sugars:** 0 g
- **Sodium:** 77 mg

3. Marinated Fish Steaks

Preparation Time: 10 minutes
Cooking Time: 15 minutes
Servings: 4
Ingredients:
- 4 lime wedges
- 2 tbsps. lime juice
- 2 minced garlic cloves
- 2 tsps. olive oil
- 1 tbsp. snipped fresh oregano
- 1 lb. fresh swordfish
- 1 tsp. lemon-pepper seasoning

Directions:
1. Rinse fish steaks; pat dry using paper towels. Cut into four serving-size pieces, if necessary.
2. In a shallow dish, put and combine lime juice, oregano, oil, lemon-pepper seasoning, and garlic. Add fish; turn to coat with marinade.
3. Cover and marinate in the refrigerator for 30 minutes to 1–1/2 hours, turning steaks occasionally. Drain fish, reserving marinade.
4. Put the fish on the greased unheated rack of a broiler pan.
5. Broil 4 inches from the heat for at least 8 to 12 minutes or until fish starts to flake when tested with a fork, turning once and brushing with reserved marinade halfway through cooking.
6. Take off any remaining marinade.
7. Before serving, squeeze the lime juice onto each steak.

Nutrition:
- **Calories:** 240
- **Fat:** 6 g
- **Carbs:** 19 g
- **Protein:** 12 g
- **Sugars:** 3.27 g
- **Sodium:** 325 mg

4. Baked Tomato Hake

Preparation Time: 10 minutes
Cooking Time: 20–25 minutes
Servings: 4
Ingredients:
- ½ cup tomato sauce
- 1 tbsp. olive oil
- a handful of parsley
- 2 sliced tomatoes
- ½ cup grated cheese
- 4 lbs. deboned and sliced hake fish
- Salt.

Directions:
1. Preheat the oven to 400°F.
2. Season the fish with salt.
3. In a skillet or saucepan, stir-fry the fish in olive oil until half-done.
4. Take four foil papers to cover the fish.
5. Shape the foil to resemble containers; add the tomato sauce into each foil container.
6. Add the fish, tomato slices, and top with grated cheese.
7. Bake until you get a golden crust for approximately 20–25 minutes.
8. Open the packs and top with parsley.

Nutrition:
- **Calories:** 265
- **Fat:** 15 g
- **Carbs:** 18 g
- **Protein:** 22 g
- **Sugars:** 0.5 g
- **Sodium:** 94.6 mg

5. Healthy Fish Nacho Bowl

Preparation Time: 13 minutes
Cooking Time: 20 minutes
Servings: 4
Ingredients:
- 500 g white fish fillets
- 400 g red cabbage
- 3 green shallots
- 1 tbsp. yogurt
- 1 tbsp. olive oil
- 425 g can black beans
- 50 g gluten-free corn chips
- 200 g cherry tomatoes
- 2–3 tsps. gluten-free chipotle seasoning
- 1 small avocado
- 1/3 cup fresh coriander leaves
- 1 large lime, rind finely grated, juiced

Directions:
1. Combine the fish, stew powder/chipotle flavoring, and 2 tsp oil in a bowl
2. Shred the cabbage in a nourishment processor fitted with the cutting connection. Move to a big bowl with the tomato, lime skin, dark beans, yogurt, 2 tbsps. lime juice, 2 shallots, and the rest of the oil. Hurl well to consolidate.
3. Heat a big non-stick skillet over high warmth. Cook the fish, turning until simply cooked through. Move to a plate.
4. Meanwhile, consolidate the avocado, coriander, remaining shallot, and 1 tbsp. remaining lime squeeze in a little bowl.
5. Divide the cabbage blend, fish, guacamole, and corn chips among serving bowls. Sprinkle with additional coriander and present with additional lime wedges.

Nutrition:
- **Calories:** 388
- **Protein:** 28.17 g
- **Fat:** 16.64 g
- **Carbs:** 35.72 g

6. Buffalo Chicken Lettuce Wraps

Preparation Time: 15 minutes
Cooking Time: 7 to 8 hours
Servings: 4
Ingredients:
1. 1 tbsp. extra virgin olive oil
2. 2 pounds boneless, skinless chicken breast
3. 2 cups vegan buffalo dip
4. 1 cup water
5. 8 to 10 romaine lettuce leaves
6. ½ red onion, thinly sliced
7. 1 cup cherry tomatoes, halved

Directions:
1. Coat the bottom of the slow cooker with olive oil.
2. Add the chicken, dip, and water, and stir to combine.
3. Cover the cooker and set it to low. Cook for around 7 to 8 hours, or until the internal temperature reaches 165°F on a meat thermometer and the juices run clear.
4. Shred the chicken using a fork, then mix it into the dip in the slow cooker.
5. Divide the meat mixture among the lettuce leaves. Top with onion and tomato, and serve.

Nutrition:
- **Calories:** 437
- **Total Fat:** 18 g
- **Total carbs:** 18 g
- **Sugar:** 8 g
- **Fiber:** 4 g
- **Protein:** 49 g
- **Sodium:** 993 mg

7. Cilantro-Lime Chicken Drumsticks

Preparation Time: 15 minutes
Cooking Time: 2 to 3 hours
Servings: 4
Ingredients:
- ¼ cup fresh cilantro, chopped
- 3 tbsps. freshly squeezed lime juice
- ½ tsp. garlic powder
- ½ tsp. sea salt
- ¼ tsp. ground cumin
- 3 pounds chicken drumsticks

Directions:
1. In a bowl, mix together the cilantro, lime juice, garlic powder, salt, and cumin to form a paste.
2. Put the drumsticks in the slow cooker. Spread the cilantro paste evenly on each drumstick.
3. Cover the cooker and set it to high. Cook for 2 to 3 hours, or until the internal temperature of the chicken reaches 165°F on a meat thermometer and the juices run clear and serve.

Nutrition:
- **Calories:** 417
- **Total Fat:** 12 g
- **Total carbs:** 1 g
- **Sugar:** 1 g
- **Fiber:** 1 g
- **Protein:** 71 g
- **Sodium:** 591 mg

8. Coconut-Curry-Cashew Chicken

Preparation Time: 15 minutes
Cooking Time: 7 to 8 hours
Servings: 4
Ingredients:
- 1 ½ cups Chicken Bone Broth
- 1 (14-oz.) can full-fat coconut milk
- 1 tsp. garlic powder
- 1 tbsp. red curry paste
- 1 tsp. sea salt
- ½ tsp. freshly ground black pepper
- ½ tsp. coconut sugar
- 2 pounds boneless, skinless chicken breasts
- 1½ cup unsalted cashews
- ½ cup diced white onion

Directions:
1. In a bowl, combine the broth, coconut milk, garlic powder, red curry paste, salt, pepper, and coconut sugar. Stir well.
2. Put the chicken, cashews, and onion in the slow cooker. Pour the coconut milk mixture on top.
3. Cover the cooker and set it to low. Cook for around 7 to 8 hours, or until the internal temperature of the chicken reaches 165°F on a meat thermometer and the juices run clear.
4. Shred the chicken using a fork, then mix it into the cooking liquid. You can also remove the chicken from the broth and chop it with a knife into bite-size pieces before returning it to the slow cooker. Serve.

Nutrition:
- **Calories:** 714
- **Total Fat:** 43 g
- **Total carbs:** 21 g
- **Sugar:** 5 g
- **Fiber:** 3 g
- **Protein:** 57 g
- **Sodium:** 1,606 mg

9. Turkey & Sweet Potato Chili

Preparation Time: 15 minutes
Cooking Time: 4 to 6 hours
Servings: 4
Ingredients:
- 1 tbsp. extra virgin olive oil
- 1 pound ground turkey
- 3 cups sweet potato cubes
- 1 (28-oz.) can diced tomatoes
- 1 red bell pepper, diced
- 1 (4-oz.) can Hatch green chiles
- ½ medium red onion, diced
- 2 cups broth of choice
- 1 tbsp. freshly squeezed lime juice
- 1 tbsp. chili powder
- 1 tsp. garlic powder
- 1 tsp. cocoa powder
- 1 tsp. ground cumin
- 1 tsp. sea salt
- ½ tsp. ground cinnamon
- Pinch cayenne pepper

Directions:
1. In your slow cooker, combine the olive oil, turkey, sweet potato cubes, tomatoes, bell pepper, chiles, onion, broth, lime juice, chili powder, garlic powder, cocoa powder, cumin, salt, cinnamon, and cayenne. Using a large spoon, break up the turkey into smaller chunks as it combines with the other ingredients.
2. Cover the cooker and set it to low. Cook for 4 to 6 hours.
3. Stir the chili well, continuing to break up the rest of the turkey, and serve.

Nutrition:
- **Calories:** 380
- **Total Fat:** 12 g
- **Total carbs:** 38 g
- **Sugar:** 12 g
- **Fiber:** 6 g
- **Protein:** 30 g
- **Sodium:** 1,268 mg

10. Moroccan Turkey Tagine

Preparation Time: 15 minutes
Cooking Time: 7 to 8 hours
Servings: 4
Ingredients:
- 4 cups boneless, skinless turkey breast chunks
- 1 (14 oz.) can diced tomatoes
- 1 (14 oz.) can chickpeas, drained
- 2 large carrots, finely chopped
- ½ cup dried apricots
- ½ red onion, chopped
- 2 tbsps. raw honey
- 1 tbsp. tomato paste
- 1 tsp. garlic powder
- 1 tsp. ground turmeric
- ½ tsp. sea salt
- ¼ tsp. ground ginger
- ¼ tsp. ground coriander
- ¼ tsp. paprika
- ½ cup water
- 2 cups broth of choice
- Freshly ground black pepper

Directions:
1. In your slow cooker, combine the turkey, tomatoes, chickpeas, carrots, apricots, onion, honey, tomato paste, garlic powder, turmeric, salt, ginger, coriander, paprika, water, and broth, and season with pepper. Gently stir to blend the ingredients.
2. Cover the cooker and set it to low. Cook for 7 to 8 hours and serve.

Nutrition:
- **Calories:** 428
- **Total Fat:** 5 g
- **Total carbs:** 46 g
- **Sugar:** 25 g
- **Fiber:** 8 g
- **Protein:** 49 g
- **Sodium:** 983 mg

11. Parsley Pork and Artichokes

Preparation Time: 10 minutes
Cooking Time: 35 minutes
Servings: 4
Ingredients:
- 2 tbsps. balsamic vinegar
- 1 cup canned artichoke hearts, drained
- 2 tbsps. olive oil
- 2 lbs. pork stew meat, cubed
- 2 tbsps. parsley, chopped
- 1 tsp. cumin, ground
- 1 tsp. turmeric powder
- 2 garlic cloves, minced
- A pinch of sea salt
- A pinch of black pepper

Directions:
1. Warm a pan with the oil on medium heat, add the meat, and brown for 5 minutes.
2. Add the artichokes, the vinegar, and the other ingredients, toss, cook over medium heat for 30 minutes, divide between plates and serve.

Nutrition:
- **Calories:** 260
- **Fat:** 5 g
- **Fiber:** 4 g
- **Carbs:** 11 g
- **Protein:** 20 g

12. Pork with Mushrooms and Cucumbers

Preparation Time: 10 minutes
Cooking Time: 25 minutes
Servings: 4
Ingredients:
- 2 tbsps. olive oil
- ½ tsp. oregano, dried
- 4 pork chops
- 2 garlic cloves, minced
- 1 lime juice
- ¼ cup cilantro, chopped
- Pinch of sea salt
- Pinch black pepper
- 1 cup white mushrooms, halved
- 2 tbsps. balsamic vinegar

Directions:
1. Warm a pan with the oil on medium heat, add the pork chops, and brown for 2 minutes on each side.
2. Put the rest of the ingredients, toss, cook on medium heat for 20 minutes, divide between plates and serve.

Nutrition:
- **Calories:** 220
- **Fat:** 6 g
- **Fiber:** 8 g
- **Carbs:** 14.2 g
- **Protein:** 20 g

13. Oregano Pork

Preparation Time: 10 minutes
Cooking Time: 8 hours
Servings: 4
Ingredients:
- 2 pounds pork roast, sliced
- 2 tbsps. oregano, chopped
- ¼ cup balsamic vinegar
- 1 cup tomato paste
- 1 tbsp. sweet paprika
- 1 tsp. onion powder
- 2 tbsps. chili powder
- 2 garlic cloves, minced
- A pinch of salt and black pepper

Directions:
1. In your slow cooker, combine the roast with the oregano, the vinegar, and the other ingredients, toss, put the lid on and cook on Low for 8 hours.
2. Divide everything between plates and serve.

Nutrition:
- **Calories:** 300
- **Fat:** 5 g
- **Fiber:** 2 g
- **Carbs:** 12 g,
- **Protein:** 24 g

14. Creamy Pork and Tomatoes

Preparation Time: 10 minutes
Cooking Time: 35 minutes
Servings: 4
Ingredients:
- 2 pounds pork stew meat, cubed
- 2 tbsps. avocado oil
- 1 cup tomatoes, cubed
- 1 cup coconut cream
- 1 tbsp. mint, chopped
- 1 jalapeño pepper, chopped
- A pinch of sea salt
- A pinch of black pepper
- 1 tbsp. hot pepper
- 2 tbsps. lemon juice

Directions:
1. Warm a pan with the oil over medium heat, add the meat, and brown for 5 minutes.
2. Add the rest of the ingredients, toss, cook over medium heat for 30 minutes more, divide between plates and serve.

Nutrition:
- **Calories:** 230
- **Fat:** 4 g
- **Fiber:** 6 g
- **Carbs:** 9 g
- **Protein:** 14 g

15. Pork with Balsamic Onion Sauce

Preparation Time: 10 minutes
Cooking Time: 35 minutes
Servings: 4
Ingredients:
- 1 yellow onion, chopped
- 4 scallions, chopped
- 2 tbsps. avocado oil
- 1 tbsp. rosemary, chopped
- 1 tbsp. lemon zest, grated
- 2 pounds pork roast, sliced
- 2 tbsps. balsamic vinegar
- ½ cup vegetable stock
- A pinch of sea salt
- A pinch of black pepper

Directions:
1. Warm a pan with the oil on medium heat, add the onion, and the scallions and sauté for 5 minutes.
2. Add the rest of the ingredients except the meat, stir, and simmer for 5 minutes.
3. Add the meat, toss gently, cook over medium heat for 25 minutes, divide between plates and serve.

Nutrition:
- **Calories:** 217
- **Fat:** 11 g
- **Fiber:** 1 g
- **Carbs:** 6 g
- **Protein:** 14 g

16. Ground Pork Pan

Preparation Time: 5 minutes
Cooking Time: 15 minutes
Servings: 4
Ingredients:
- 2 garlic cloves, minced
- 2 red chilies, chopped
- 2 tbsps. olive oil
- 2 pounds pork stew meat, ground
- 1 red bell pepper, chopped
- 1 green bell pepper, chopped
- 1 tomato, cubed
- ½ cup mushrooms, halved
- Pinch of sea salt
- Pinch black pepper
- 1 tbsp. basil, chopped
- 2 tbsps. coconut aminos

Directions:
1. Warm a pan with the oil on medium heat, add the garlic, chilies, bell peppers, tomato, and mushrooms and sauté for 5 minutes.
2. Add the meat and the rest of the ingredients, toss, cook over medium heat for 10 minutes more, divide between plates and serve.

Nutrition:
- **Calories:** 200
- **Fat:** 3 g
- **Fiber:** 5 g
- **Carbs:** 7 g
- **Protein:** 17 g

17. Fish & Chickpea Stew

Preparation Time: 5 minutes
Cooking Time: 10 minutes
Servings: 4
Ingredients:
- 2 cups fish stock
- 1 brown onion
- 400 g can tomatoes
- 4 kale leaves
- 500 g firm white fish fillets
- 1 pc. sliced coles bakery stone
- 2 garlic cloves
- Finely grated parmesan, to serve (as desired)
- 400 g can chickpeas
- 1 carrot, peeled
- Salt and pepper to taste

Directions:
1. Spray a skillet with an olive oil shower. Spot over medium-low warmth. Include the carrot and onion and cook, mixing, until delicate and brilliant. Include garlic and cook, blending until sweet-smelling.
2. Add the chickpeas stock and tomato, and to the onion blend in the skillet. Bring to the bubble. Lessen warmth to medium-low and stew until the blend thickens somewhat.
3. Add the kale and fish to the dish and stew until the fish is simply cooked through. Season.
4. Divide the stew among serving bowls. Sprinkle with parmesan and present with the bread.

Nutrition:
- **Calories:** 1447
- **Protein:** 42.1 g
- **Fat:** 127.85 g
- **Carbs:** 32.4 g

18. Duck Legs and Wine Sauce

Preparation Time: 10 minutes
Cooking Time: 1 hour and 30 minutes
Servings: 4
Ingredients:
- 4 duck legs, trimmed
- Salt and black pepper
- 1 tsp. olive oil
- 2 shallots, chopped
- 1 carrot, chopped
- 1 ½ cups red wine
- 2 tsps. tomato paste
- ½ cup chicken stock
- 2 tbsps. sugar
- 1 tbsp. balsamic vinegar
- 1 tsp. rosemary, dried

Directions:
1. Warm a pan with the oil on medium-high heat.
2. Add duck legs, season with salt and pepper, brown for 5 minutes on all sides, and transfer to a plate.
3. Heat the same pan over medium heat, add the shallots and carrots, stir and cook for 2 minutes.
4. Add the wine, tomato paste, stock, sugar, vinegar, rosemary, stir and simmer for 5 minutes.
5. Return the duck legs, toss, cook everything for 1 hour and 30 over medium-low heat stirring often, divide everything between plates and serve.

Nutrition:
- **Calories:** 257
- **Fat:** 14 g
- **Fiber:** 6 g
- **Carbs:** 14 g
- **Protein:** 8 g

19. Chicken Piccata

Preparation Time: 15 minutes
Cooking Time: 30 minutes
Servings: 4
Ingredients:
- 4 boneless, skinless chicken breast
- 1 cup ground almond meal
- 1/4 cup grated Parmesan cheese
- 1/2 tsp. Dijon mustard
- 1 yellow onion, chopped
- 1 tsp. sea salt
- 1/2 tsp. ground black pepper
- 4 tbsps. olive oil
- 4 tbsps. organic unsalted butter
- 1/2 cup organic, gluten-free chicken broth
- 3 tbsps. lemon juice
- 2 tbsps. capers
- 3 tbsps. organic butter
- 1/4 cup fresh parsley, chopped

Directions:
1. Combine the almond meal, cheese, mustard, salt, and pepper spread the mixture on a shallow dish.
2. Wash the pounded chicken breasts in water and shake off the excess. Dredge the chicken in the flour mixture.
3. Add tbsps. of butter in a large saucepan over high heat; add the olive oil.
4. Cook chicken in butter and oil for approximately 3–4 minutes on each side until golden brown.
5. Place the cooked chicken on a serving dish and cover it to keep warm.
6. Stir in the chicken broth, lemon juice, and capers, scraping up any brown bits in the pan. Add the chicken broth, lemon juice, and capers to the skillet, stirring and scraping up any brown bits in the skillet. Simmer until the sauce is reduced and reaches a light syrup consistency. Reduce heat to low and stir in remaining butter.
7. Ladle the sauce over the chicken breasts and top with chopped parsley. Serve with lemon slices or wedges.

Nutrition:
- **Calories:** 357 **Protein:** 4.51 g **Fat:** 35.73 g **Carbs:** 6.16 g

20. Honey-Mustard Lemon Marinated Chicken

Preparation Time: 10 minutes
Cooking Time: 20 minutes
Servings: 4
Ingredients:
- 1 pound lean chicken breast
- 1/4 cup Dijon mustard
- 1 tbsp. olive oil
- 1/4 cup rosemary leaves, chopped
- 1 lemon, zested and juiced
- 1 tbsp. cayenne pepper
- 1/2 tsp. ground black pepper
- 1/2 tsp. sea salt

Directions:
1. Place chicken breasts in a 7x11-inch baking dish.
2. Mix together all ingredients except the chicken in a medium bowl.
3. Pour prepared marinade over chicken; turn sides to coat. Cover, place in the fridge, and marinate for an hour or overnight for the best flavor.
4. Bake at 350°F for 20 minutes.
5. Use the extra sauce over the top and serve.

Nutrition:
- **Calories:** 265
- **Protein:** 26.12 g
- **Fat:** 16.27 g
- **Carbs:** 3.08 g

21. Easy Crunchy Fish Tray Bake

Preparation Time: 10 minutes
Cooking Time: 20 minutes
Servings: 4
Ingredients:
- 600 g frozen crumbed whiting fish fillets
- 1/2 small red onion
- 2 x 250 g punnets tomatoes
- 2 zucchini
- 180 g baby stuffed peppers
- 1 tbsp. parmesan
- 2 tsps. oregano leaves
- 1 lemon, cut into wedges

Directions:
1. Preheat the oven to 400°F. Oil a big preparing plate. Spot the fish filets on the readied plate. Disperse the oregano and parmesan over the fish.
2. Add the zucchini, tomatoes, and stuffed peppers to the plate. Disperse the onion rings over the top. Season well. Splash with olive oil. Heat until the fish is brilliant and cooked through.
3. Divide the fish and vegetables among plates and present with the rocket and lemon wedges.

Nutrition:
- **Calories:** 346
- **Protein:** 3.67 g
- **Fat:** 2.8 g
- **Carbs:** 81.77 g

22. Ginger & Chili Sea Bass Fillets

Preparation Time: 5 minutes
Cooking Time: 10 minutes
Servings: 2
Ingredients:
- 2 sea bass fillet
- 1 tsp. black pepper
- 1 tbsp. extra virgin olive oil
- 1 tsp. ginger, peeled and chopped
- 1 garlic clove, thinly sliced
- 1 red chili, deseeded and thinly sliced
- 2 green onions stemmed, chopped

Directions:
1. Get a skillet and heat the oil on medium to high heat.
2. Sprinkle black pepper over the Sea Bass and score the fish's skin a few times with a sharp knife.
3. Add the sea bass fillet to the very hot pan with the skin side down.
4. Cook for 5 minutes and turn over.
5. Cook for a further 2 minutes.
6. Remove sea bass from the pan and rest.
7. Put the chili, garlic, and ginger and cook for approximately 2 minutes or until golden.
8. Remove from the heat and add the green onions.
9. Scatter the vegetables over your sea bass to serve.
10. Try with a steamed sweet potato or side salad.

Nutrition:
- **Calories:** 306
- **Protein:** 29.92 g
- **Fat:** 8.94 g
- **Carbs:** 26.59 g

23. Cheesy Tuna Pasta

Preparation Time: 10 minutes
Cooking Time: 20 minutes
Servings: 2-4
Ingredients:
- 2 cups arugula
- ¼ cup chopped green onions
- 1 tbs. red vinegar
- 5 oz. drained canned tuna
- ¼ tsp. black pepper
- 2 oz. cooked whole-wheat pasta
- 1 tbsp. olive oil
- 1 tbsp. grated low-fat parmesan

Directions:
1. Cook the pasta in unsalted water until ready. Drain and set aside.
2. In a large-sized bowl, thoroughly mix the tuna, green onions, vinegar, oil, arugula, pasta, and black pepper.
3. Toss well and top with the cheese.
4. Serve and enjoy.

Nutrition:
- **Calories:** 566.3
- **Fat:** 42.4 g
- **Carbs:** 18.6 g
- **Protein:** 29.8 g
- **Sugars:** 0.4 g
- **Sodium:** 688.6 mg

24. Salmon and Roasted Peppers

Preparation Time: 5 minutes
Cooking Time: 25 minutes
Servings: 4
Ingredients:
- 1 cup red peppers, cut into strips
- 4 salmon fillets, boneless
- ¼ cup chicken stock
- 2 tbsps. olive oil
- 1 yellow onion, chopped
- 1 tbsp. cilantro, chopped
- A pinch of sea salt
- A pinch of black pepper

Directions:
1. Warm a pan with the oil on medium-high heat; add the onion and sauté for 5 minutes.
2. Put the fish and cook for at least 5 minutes on each side.
3. Add the rest of the ingredients, introduce the pan in the oven, and cook at 390°F for 10 minutes.
4. Divide the mix between plates and serve.

Nutrition:
- **Calories:** 265
- **Fat:** 7 g
- **Fiber:** 5 g
- **Carbs:** 15 g
- **Protein:** 16 g

CHAPTER 5:

Desserts

1. Chocolate Chip Quinoa Granola Bars

Preparation Time: 5 minutes
Cooking Time: 10 minutes
Servings: 16
Ingredients:
- ½ cup chia seeds
- ½ cup walnuts, chopped
- 1 cup buckwheat
- 1 cup uncooked quinoa
- 2/3 cup dairy-free margarine
- ½ cup flaxseed
- 1 tsp. cinnamon
- ½ cup honey
- ½ cup chocolate chips
- 1 tsp. vanilla
- ¼ tsp. salt

Directions:
1. Preheat your oven to 350°F.
2. Spread the walnuts, quinoa, wheat, flaxseed, and chia on your baking sheet.
3. Bake for 10 minutes.
4. Line your baking dish with plastic wrap. Apply cooking spray. Keep aside.
5. Melt the margarine and honey in a saucepot.
6. Whisk together the vanilla, salt, and cinnamon into the margarine mix.
7. Keep the wheat mix and quinoa in a bowl. Pour the margarine sauce into it.
8. Stir the mixture. Coat well. Allow it to cool. Stir in the chocolate chips.
9. Spread your mixture into the baking dish. Press firmly into the pan.
10. Plastic wrap. Refrigerator overnight.
11. Slice into bars and serve.

Nutrition:
- **Calories:** 408 **Carbohydrates:** 31 g **Fat:** 28 g **Protein:** 8 g **Sugar:** 14 g
- **Fiber:** 6 g **Sodium:** 87mg

2. Sherbet Pineapple

Preparation Time: 20 minutes
Cooking Time: 0 minutes
Servings: 4
Ingredients:
- 1 can (8-oz.) pineapple chunks
- 1/3 cup orange marmalade
- ¼ tsp. ground ginger
- ¼ tsp. vanilla extract
- 1 can (11-oz.) orange sections
- 2 cups pineapple, lemon, or lime sherbet

Directions:
1. Drain the pineapple, ensure you reserve the juice.
2. Take a medium-sized bowl and add pineapple juice, ginger, vanilla, and marmalade to the bowl
3. Add pineapple chunks, drained mandarin oranges as well
4. Toss well and coat everything
5. Free them for 15 minutes and allow them to chill
6. Spoon the sherbet into 4 chilled stemmed sherbet dishes
7. Top each of them with the fruit mixture
8. Enjoy!

Nutrition:
- **Calories:** 267 Cal
- **Fat:** 1 g
- **Carbs:** 65 g
- **Protein:** 2 g

3. Easy Peach Cobbler

Preparation Time: 5 minutes
Cooking Time: 20 minutes
Servings: 6
Ingredients:
- 5 organic peaches, pitted and chopped
- ¼ cup coconut palm sugar, divided
- ½ tsp. cinnamon
- ¾ cup chopped pecans
- ½ cup gluten-free oats
- ¼ cup ground flaxseeds
- ¼ brown rice flour
- ¼ cup extra virgin olive oil

Directions:
1. Preheat the oven to 350°F.
2. Grease the bottom of 6 ramekins.
3. In a bowl, mix the peaches, ½ of the coconut sugar, cinnamon, and pecans.
4. Distribute the peach mixture into the ramekins.
5. In the same bowl, mix the oats, flaxseed, rice flour, and oil. Add in the remaining coconut sugar. Mix until a crumbly texture is formed.
6. Top the mixture over the peaches.
7. Set for 20 minutes.

Nutrition:
- Calories 26
- **Fat:** 11 g
- **Carbs:** 28 g
- **Protein:** 10 g
- **Sugar:** 12 g
- **Fiber:** 6 g

4. Thar She Salts Peanut Butter Cookies

Preparation Time: 15 minutes
Cooking Time: 0 minutes
Servings: 9
Ingredients:
- 1 cup raw almonds
- ½ a cup peanut butter (creamy and unsalted)
- 1 cup pitted Medjool dates
- 1 ¼ tsp. vanilla extract
- Sea salt as needed

Directions:
1. Take a food processor and add almonds, peanut butter, vanilla, dates and blend the whole mixture until a dough-like texture comes (should take a few minutes).
2. If you want, add some more peanut butter to make the dough sticker.
3. Form balls using the dough and press down using a fork to create a criss-cross pattern.
4. Sprinkle salt generously.
5. Serve immediately.

Nutrition:
- **Calories:** 350
- **Fat:** 17 g
- **Carbs:** 27 g
- **Protein:** 18 g

5. Fruit Cobbler

Preparation Time: 10 minutes
Cooking Time: 20 minutes
Servings: 8
Ingredients:
- 1 tsp. coconut oil
- ¼ cup coconut oil, melted
- 2 cups peaches, fresh & sliced
- 2 cups nectarines, fresh & sliced
- 2 tbsps. lemon juice, fresh
- ¾ cup rolled oats
- ¾ cup almond flour
- ¼ cup coconut sugar
- ½ tsp. vanilla extract, pure
- 1 tsp. ground cinnamon
- A dash salt
- Filter water for mixing

Directions:
1. Start by heating your oven to 425°F.
2. Get out a cast-iron skillet, coating it with a tsp. of coconut oil.
3. Mix your lemon juice, peaches, and nectarines together in the skillet.
4. Get out a food processor, mixing your almond flour, oats, coconut sugar, and remaining coconut oil. Add in your cinnamon, vanilla, and salt, pulsing until the oat mixture resembles a dry dough.
5. If you need more moisture, add filtered water a tbsp. at a time, and then break the dough into chunks, spreading it across the fruit.
6. Bake for twenty minutes before serving warm.

Nutrition:
- **Protein:** 4 g
- **Fat:** 12 g
- **Carbs:** 15 g

6. Watermelon and Avocado Cream

Preparation Time: 2 hours
Cooking Time: 0 minutes
Servings: 4
Ingredients:
- 2 cups coconut cream
- 1 watermelon, peeled and chopped
- 2 avocados, peeled, pitted and chopped
- 1 tbsp. honey
- 2 tsps. lemon juice

Directions:
1. In a blender, put all the ingredients. Divide it into bowls and keep it in the fridge for 2 hours before serving.

Nutrition:
- **Calories:** 121
- **Fat:** 2 g
- **Fiber:** 2 g
- **Carbs:** 6 g
- **Protein:** 5 g

7. Coconut and Chocolate Cream

Preparation Time: 2 hours
Cooking Time: 0 minutes
Servings: 4
Ingredients:
- 2 cups coconut milk
- 2 tbsps. ginger, grated
- 2 tbsps. honey
- 1 cup dark chocolate, chopped and melted
- ½ tsp. cinnamon powder
- 1 tsp. vanilla extract

Directions:
1. In a blender, put all the ingredients and blend. Divide into bowls and place in the fridge for 2 hours before serving.

Nutrition:
- **Calories:** 200
- **Fat:** 3 g
- **Fiber:** 5 g
- **Carbs:** 12 g
- **Protein:** 7 g

8. Chocolate Bananas

Preparation Time: 5 minutes
Cooking Time: 15 minutes
Servings: 4
Ingredients:
- 3 bananas, large and cut into thirds
- 12 oz. dark chocolate
- 1 tbsp. coconut oil

Directions:
2. Melt the chocolate and coconut oil in a double boiler for 3 to 4 minutes, till you get a smooth and glossy mixture.
3. Next, keep the popsicles at the end of each of the bananas by inserting them.
4. After that, immerse the chocolate into the warm chocolate mixture.
5. Shake off the excess chocolate and place them on parchment paper.
6. Sprinkle with the topping of your choice.
7. Finally, place them in the freezer for a few hours or until set.
8. Tip: You can use topping like chopped pistachios or with unsweetened chocolate sprinkles, etc.

Nutrition:
- **Calories:** 427
- Proteins: 5.9 g
- **Carbs:** 80 g
- **Fat:** 15.6 g

9. Watermelon Sorbet

Preparation Time: 5 minutes
Cooking Time: 15 minutes
Servings: 4
Ingredients:
- 1 Seedless Watermelon, cubed

Directions:
1. To start with, place the watermelon cubes in a baking sheet in an even layer.
2. After that, keep the sheet in the freezer for 2 hours or until the watermelon is solid.
3. Next, transfer the frozen watermelon cubes to the high-speed blender and puree them until you get a smooth puree.
4. Then pour the puree among the two loaf pans.

Nutrition:
- **Calories:** 427
- **Proteins:** 5.9 g
- **Carbs:** 80 g
- **Fat:** 15.6 g

10. Almond Butter Balls Vegan

Preparation Time: 10 minutes
Cooking Time: 0 minutes
Servings: 4
Ingredients:
- 12 dates, pitted and diced
- 1/3 cup unsweetened shredded coconut
- 2 ½ tbsp. almond butter

Directions:
1. Take a bowl and add dates, almond butter, and coconut.
2. Mix well.
3. Use the mixture to form small balls.
4. Store them in your fridge and chill them.
5. Enjoy!

Nutrition:
- **Calories:** 62
- **Fats:** 3 g
- **Carbs:** 8 g
- **Protein:** 1 g

11. Coffee Cream

Preparation Time: 10 minutes
Cooking Time: 15 minutes
Servings: 4
Ingredients:
- ¼ cup brewed coffee
- 2 tbsps. swerve
- 2 cups heavy cream
- 1 tsp. vanilla extract
- 2 tbsps. ghee, melted
- 2 eggs

Directions:
1. In a bowl, combine the coffee with the cream and the other ingredients, whisk well and divide it into 4 ramekins and whisk well.
2. Introduce the ramekins in the oven at 350°F and bake for 15 minutes.
3. Serve warm.

Nutrition:
- **Calories:** 300
- **Fat:** 11 g
- **Carbs:** 3 g
- **Protein:** 4 g
- **Sugar:** 12 g

12. Almond Cookies

Preparation Time: 15 minutes
Cooking Time: 15 minutes
Servings: 12
Ingredients:
- 14 oz./400 g non-wheat flour
- 1 tsp. baking soda
- 1 tsp. baking powder
- 3.5 oz./100 g tahini
- 1.7 oz./50 g coconut butter
- ½ tsp. vanilla
- ½ tsp. honey
- Salt

Directions:
1. Mix the flour, soda, salt, baking powder together.
2. Mix tahini and coconut butter together and add 2 tbsp. water to the same bowl.
3. Add honey, vanilla to the tahini mixture and blend it well with a mixer.
4. Preheat your oven (180°C/356°F) and put a baking sheet on it.
5. Add 24 tbsps. of the mixture onto the baking sheet and let it bake in the oven for 11–15 minutes.
6. Let it get cold a little bit and serve.

Nutrition:
- **Calories:** 112
- **Carbs:** 18 g
- **Protein:** 3.2 g
- **Fat:** 1.6 g
- **Sugar:** 23.1 g
- **Fiber:** 7.4 g
- **Sodium:** 28 mg

13. Chocolate Mousse

Preparation Time: 10 minutes
Cooking Time: 0 minutes
Servings: 4
Ingredients:
- Coconut cream scraped from the upper side of 2 pieces of 13.5-ounce chilled cans of full-fat coconut milk
- 4 tbsps. cocoa
- 3 tbsps. Agave Nectar
- 1 tsp. vanilla extract

Directions:
1. Take a large bowl and scoop out the thick coconut cream from the can to the bowl
2. Add nectar, vanilla extract, and cocoa to the bowl
3. Beat it well using an electric mixer, starting from low and going to medium until a foamy texture appears
4. Divide the mix evenly amongst ramekins and chill to your desired level of cold
5. Enjoy!

Nutrition:
- **Calories:** 134
- **Fat:** 3.8 g
- **Carbs:** 16 g
- **Protein:** 3.8 g

14. Strawberry Granita

Preparation Time: 10 minutes
Cooking Time: 10 minutes
Servings: 8
Ingredients:
- 2 lbs. strawberries, halved & hulled
- 1 cup water
- Agave to taste
- ¼ tsp. balsamic vinegar
- ½ tsp. lemon juice
- Just a small pinch of salt

Directions:
1. Rinse the strawberries in water.
2. Keep in a blender. Add water, agave, balsamic vinegar, salt, and lemon juice.
3. Pulse many times so that the mixture moves. Blend to make it smooth.
4. Pour into a baking dish. The puree should be 3/8 inch deep only.
5. Refrigerate the dish uncovered until the edges start to freeze. The center should be slushy.
6. Stir crystals from the edges lightly into the center. Mix thoroughly.
7. Chill till the granite is almost completely frozen.
8. Scrape loose the crystals like before and mix.
9. Refrigerate again. Use a fork to stir 3–4 times until the granite has become light.

Nutrition:
- **Calories:** 72
- **Carbs:** 17 g
- **Fat:** 0 g
- **Sugar:** 14 g
- **Fiber:** 2 g
- **Protein:** 1 g

15. Apple Fritters

Preparation Time: 15 minutes
Cooking Time: 10 minutes
Servings: 4
Ingredients:
- 1 apple, cored, peeled, and chopped
- 1 cup all-purpose flour
- 1 egg
- ½ cup cashew milk
- 1–1/2 tsp. baking powder
- 2 tbsps. of stevia

Directions:
1. Preheat your air fryer to 175°C or 350°F.
2. Keep parchment paper at the bottom of your fryer.
3. Apply cooking spray.
4. Mix together ¼ cup sugar, flour, baking powder, egg, milk, and salt in a bowl.
5. Combine well by stirring.
6. Sprinkle 2 tbsps. of sugar on the apples. Coat well.
7. Combine the apples with your flour mixture.
8. Use a cookie scoop and drop the fritters with it to the air fryer basket's bottom.
9. Now air fry for 5 minutes.
10. Flip the fritters once and fry for another 3 minutes. They should be golden.

Nutrition:
- **Calories:** 307
- **Carbohydrates:** 65 g
- **Cholesterol:** 48 mg
- **Total Fat:** 3 g
- **Protein:** 5 g
- **Sugar:** 39 g
- **Fiber:** 2 g
- **Sodium:** 248mg

Conclusion

Thank you for making it through to the end of the "Anti-Inflammatory Diet Cookbook." Let's hope it was informative and able to provide you with all the tools you must attain your goals, whatever they may be. Inflammation is a normal process of our immune system and completely necessary to protect us from threats that will damage our cells and tissues. If it weren't for our immune system, our bodies would be ravaged instantly by deadly diseases, and the results would be fatal. As long as the inflammatory process does not last beyond its normal time, there is usually no issue. Once the inflammation becomes chronic or long-term, it becomes an inflammatory disease and will create damaging results.

The inflammatory disease will lead to many different health consequences and will even attack our most vital organs. The best way to do this is to prevent chronic inflammation in the first place. The next best thing is to recognize the signs and symptoms as early as possible, so proper interventions can be done to limit and reverse the impact of chronic inflammation. Inflammatory disease is the root cause of many long-term diseases, so ignoring the warning signs can create major consequences for your health.

Unfortunately, if the inflammatory disease gets out of control, preventative measures may be out of the question, and medical interventions will need to be done. Our goal is to prevent you from getting to this point. Lucky for us, many lifestyle changes can be performed to stop and reverse this disease process when it is still in its advanced stages. This is another reason why we should recognize and not ignore the signs and symptoms. A major lifestyle change we can commit to is a new diet plan. The anti-inflammatory diet is a meal plan that boasts healthy and nutritious cuisines, but still flavorful and appealing to the taste buds. There is a major myth out there that healthy food cannot be delicious. We have proven this myth wrong by providing numerous recipes from around the world that follow our healthy meal plan.

We hope that the information you read in this book gives you a better understanding of how the immune system functions and how a proper diet plan can help protect it and our other valuable cells and tissues. The recipes we have provided are just a starting point. Use them as a guide to create many of your dishes that follow the diet plan. Just make sure you use the proper ingredients and food groups. Also, for maximum results, follow the "Anti-Inflammatory Diet food Guide Pyramid."

The next step is to take the instruction we have provided and begin taking steps to change your life and improve your health. Begin recognizing the signs and symptoms of chronic inflammation and make the necessary lifestyle changes to prevent further health problems. Start transitioning to the anti-inflammatory diet today by incorporating small meals into your schedule and increase the amount as tolerated.

Within a short period, the diet will be a regular part of your routine. You will notice increased energy, improved mental function, a stronger and well-balanced immune system, reduction in chronic pain, some healthy weight loss, and overall better health outcomes. If you are ready to experience these changes, then wait no longer and begin putting your knowledge from this book into action.